Advanced Medical Nutrition Therapy Practice

Annalynn Skipper, PhD, RD, FADA
Author
Consultant
Oak Park, IL

JONES AND BARTLETT PUBLISHERS
Sudbury, Massachusetts
BOSTON   TORONTO   LONDON   SINGAPORE

World Headquarters

Jones and Bartlett Publishers
40 Tall Pine Drive
Sudbury, MA 01776
978-443-5000
info@jbpub.com
www.jbpub.com

Jones and Bartlett Publishers
Canada
6339 Ormindale Way
Mississauga, Ontario L5V 1J2
CANADA

Jones and Bartlett Publishers
International
Barb House, Barb Mews
London W6 7PA
United Kingdom

Jones and Bartlett's books and products are available through most bookstores and online booksellers. To contact Jones and Bartlett Publishers directly, call 800-832-0034, fax 978-443-8000, or visit our website, www.jbpub.com.

Substantial discounts on bulk quantities of Jones and Bartlett's publications are available to corporations, professional associations, and other qualified organizations. For details and specific discount information, contact the special sales department at Jones and Bartlett via the above contact information or send an email to specialsales@jbpub.com.

This publication is designed to provide accurate and authoritative information in regard to the Subject Matter covered. It is sold with the understanding that the publisher is not engaged in rendering legal, accounting, or other professional service. If legal advice or oher expert assistance is required, the service of a competent professional person should be sought.

Production Credits

Publisher: Michael Brown
Production Director: Amy Rose
Associate Editor: Katey Birtcher
Production Editor: Tracey Chapman
Marketing Manager: Wendy Thayer
Manufacturing Buyer: Therese Connell
Composition: Publishers' Design and Production Services, Inc.
Cover Design: Kristin E. Ohlin
Printing and Binding: Malloy, Inc.
Cover Printing: Malloy, Inc.
Cover Image: © Bidouze Stéphane/ShutterStock, Inc.

Library of Congress Cataloging-in-Publication Data

Skipper, Annalynn.
    Advanced medical nutrition therapy practice / Annalynn Skipper.—1st ed.
      p. ; cm.
Includes bibliographical references and index.
    ISBN 978-0-7637-4289-8 (alk. paper)
    1. Diet therapy. 2. Dietetics—Practice. I. Title.
    [DNLM: 1. Nutrition Therapy—methods. 2. Models, Theoretical. 3. Professional Practice.
WB 400 S628a 2008]
    RM216.S545 2008
    615.8′54—dc22

2007028617

6048

Printed in the United States of America
12 11 10 09 08   10 9 8 7 6 5 4 3 2 1

Contents

List of Figures, Tables, and Exhibits

FIGURES

TABLES

EXHIBITS

Acknowledgments

This text is a composite of thinking that has been shaped during years of practice, teaching, research, and my own education. Several of my fellow graduate students and colleagues at Texas Tech helped me understand what it meant to read the literature and think about how I practiced. The faculty there, especially Margarette Hardin, Clara McPherson, and Mina Lamb, were patient teachers and effective mentors.

My colleague Anne Marie Hunter has endured and contributed to discussions about advanced practice for more than two decades. Jennifer Nelson and others who served with me on the ASPEN Dietitian's Committee have also intermittently participated in an ongoing discourse about advanced practice that began when we developed the CNSD credential. Several of my colleagues at Hahneman Hospital, Pennsylvania Hospital, and other Philadelphia institutions spent long days on the beach discussing dietetics practice with me. In Chicago, I have been privileged to work with several accomplished nutrition support dietitians. My attempts to obtain appropriate compensation for their skills, while ultimately unsuccessful, was the impetus for this attempt to define what it is that advanced practice dietitians do.

I have been privileged to learn a great deal about expertise from colleagues in medicine and nursing. The surgical residents at the Pennsylvania Hospital shared astute observations of mature practice that helped me to understand that much remains to be learned after formal education is complete. Also, at the Pennsylvania Hospital, I had the privilege to have David Paskin, who was expertise personified, as a mentor. Keith Millikan, with whom I co-directed the Nutrition Support Service at Rush University Medical Center, provided a wonderful example of clinical teaching. Ellen Elpern, Margaret Faut-Callahan, and Martha Siomos at Rush University each taught me a great deal about advanced practice nursing. Their courses and practice played a major role in my research.

This book exists because I decided to complete a PhD at the University of Nebraska, several hundred miles from my home in a Chicago suburb. Joann Carson made that degree attainable for me when she shared her experiences with air commuting. She made me realize that I could fly to class in Lincoln. Joanne was also there at the end of my PhD when she ably chaired American Society of Nutrition Sciences Meeting where I presented the results of my research. While I was in school, my staff and a few of my colleagues at Rush University provided much appreciated encouragement, especially Sally Lipson, Mary Spooner, and Diana Barry.

Nebraska is a quiet, peaceful place with vast spaces that nurture great thinkers. There I was privileged to work with Jim King, Linda Boeckner, and Kay Stanek-Krogstrand. The nutrition classes at the University of Nebraska were of the highest order, especially those related to nutrition diagnosis, nutrition pharmacology, and evidence analysis, but I learned a great deal outside of nutrition as well. Lloyd Bell helped me think creatively about educational techniques. Gerald Parsons provided many wonderful insights into leadership and how it might apply outside of the classical sense. Ron Shope taught me the qualitative research methods that were refined in a New York class with Sharlene Hesse-Biber. Charles Ansorge taught me, a lifelong mathophobe, to do meaningful statistical analysis. Kent Eskridge provided statistical support to my project. All of these individuals influenced the breadth of thinking necessary to create an advanced practice model. Of course, I would never have started or finished this effort without Nancy Lewis, my research mentor and major professor. Her insights and thoughtful questions made major contributions to my research. I am grateful for the patience, time, and insights that she brought to this project.

Beverly Mitchell at the Commission on Accreditation of Dietetic Education has taught me a great deal about dietetic education as have members of the Accreditation Standards Committee, especially Linda Young, Louise Peck, and Marsha Pfeiffer. Many ideas about education were developed and tested during conversations with my colleagues on the Dietetic Education Task Force. Charlette Gallagher Allred, Patsy Brannon, Cathy Wotecki, Bob Earl, Constance Geiger, Karen Greathouse, Leslene Gordon, Ellen Owens Summo, Sue Lesson, David Orozco, Glenda Price, Evelyn Enrione, Yolanda Ortega-Gammill, Riva Touger-Decker, Marsha Schofield, and Harold Hollar stimulated my thinking about advanced practice education.

Wanda Hain Howell and Sally Ann Henry mentored my entry into the realm of credentialing when I was part of the group developing the Certified Nutrition Support Dietitian (CNSD) certificate. A few years later, Joanne Wade, Michael

Kane, and Carmen Estes provided a different perspective on credentialing as we worked on the Metabolic Nutrition Care credential. Chris Reidy at the Commission on Dietetic Registration has helped me to clarify my thinking about the difference in specialty and advanced credentials. My colleagues on the advanced practice audit committee, Judy Fish, Bill Barkley, JoAnne Cassell, Doris Fredericks, Constance Geiger, Joyce Gilbert, Karmeen Kulkarni, Martha Lynch, Penny McConnell, Charles Mueller, Esther Myers, Janet Skates, Kay Manger-Hague, and Dick Rogers have engaged in spirited dialogue that has shaped my thinking about an advanced practice credential.

I am grateful to Karren Moreland, Heidi Silver, Deborah Wildish, and especially Mary Hager who broadened my perspective on order writing and autonomous practice. Karen Lacey and Carolyn Cochran furthered my thinking about models. Esther Myers encouraged me to clearly describe advanced practice so that it could be differentiated from basic practice. Julie O'Sullivan Maillet, Charlene Compher, Nancy Hakel-Smith, and Jean Guest reacted to some very early drafts of exhibits. Janet Skates and Trisha Furhman commented on later ones. Pam Charney, Trisha Fuhrman, Mary Russell, Ainsley Malone, and Mary Marian provided immediate and thoughtful feedback on many ideas. Ruth DeBusk, Laura Matarese, Linda Snetselaar, and Sandy Austhoff shared expertise in their areas of practice. The many dietitians, some from other countries, who have called or e-mailed with questions and comments that stimulated my thinking about how we practice are an important stimulus for this book. It is impossible to express my gratitude to the very busy, accomplished and expert advanced practice dietitians that participated in the study that supports the model. These accomplished dietitians confirmed that advanced practice in dietetics not only exists, but can be described. Confidentiality prohibits me from thanking them by name for their inspirational words.

This book would not exist without Mike Brown at Jones and Bartlett who has encouraged, cajoled, and sometimes begged me to finish the four books we have done together. Katey Birtcher, Jennifer Ryan, and Jill Hobbs have done an excellent job of editing this work. I am incredibly fortunate to have such an impressive group of colleagues. If I have misinterpreted their insights, advice, and teaching, I apologize and accept responsibility for the flaws in this book.

Of course I'm grateful to my family and friends who encouraged me while I developed the ideas in this text. I am especially grateful to Louise Skipper, Ellen Skipper, and Matt and Megan Smith. This book is dedicated to Joe Smith who has been there from start to finish and enjoyed it all so much. Thanks Joe, for the dinner table conversations, the use of your extensive library, and the lunchbox!

Preface

Many clinical dietitians know an outstanding preceptor, mentor, or colleague who practices at an advanced level. These advanced practice dietitians often use exceptional knowledge and skill to obtain superior outcomes. Patients and colleagues alike seek this dietitian's expertise. They easily and willingly teach others, automatically sensing the appropriate level of information to provide. When faced with problems, challenges, or changes in the healthcare system, these dietitians offer optimism, innovation, and creativity. When new information becomes available they may lead in implementing it but may also reject it because it is scientifically unsound. This dietitian is often invited to collaborate with others, and frequently participates in multidisciplinary efforts.

At the same time, there are many dietitians with decades of experience that practice at a basic level. These dietitians are content to follow the trends, letting others lead the way. They are the implementers, the worker bees. They provide good, solid medical nutrition therapy day in and day out. They are the backbone of the dietetics profession. They are by far the majority. They are much needed.

The same situation exists in other professions; in nursing, in medicine, in law, and in philosophy. Some distinguish themselves by leading practice, and others prefer to follow. In other professions there are outlets for these top tier individuals. In medicine and law, they may build a successful practice or firm. In philosophy, they may obtain academic promotion or develop a consulting practice. In nursing, there is a clearly defined career path to advanced practice positions. Licensure and other laws govern advanced nursing practice. Educational programs support advanced practice nurses. Salary schedules are designed to attract and retain advanced practice nurses in hospitals and clinics.

In dietetics, we are taught that career advancement is only available in management or in academia. Yet few dietitians with an interest in medical nutrition therapy wish to change to another field such as education or administration. At the same time, patient care is becoming more and more complex. As we recall what we have learned or taught ourselves during our careers, it is clear that medical nutrition therapy is complex enough to support advanced level practice.

As we encounter advanced practice dietitians, we have many questions. What exactly is advanced dietetics practice? What skills are needed to practice at an advanced level? How do advanced practice dietitians acquire their skills? Do they have special knowledge, or unique experiences or training in their background? Is it possible to train advanced practice dietitians? What skills does the advanced practice dietitian have that an employer will value and reward? These questions have concerned me for more than two decades, and these are the questions that this book will explore.

This is not a book filled with facts, formulas, "secrets," or "clinical pearls." The absence of this type of information may be a disappointment to many. Instead of the "checklist" approach to achieving advanced practice status, this book contains a collection of ideas as a single advanced practice theory. This book is not a recipe for advanced practice, but an explanation of ideas about what an advanced practice dietitian does differently from a specialist or basic level practitioner. Hopefully, this theory provides a framework that will engender discussion and debate. Nothing would make me happier.

CHAPTER 1

Advanced Medical Nutrition Therapy Practice: An Introduction and Rationale

"Without rungs on the ladder, there is nowhere to climb."

Intuitively, we know that advanced medical nutrition therapy practice exists. Most dietitians can identify at least one professional colleague who is beyond others in providing patient care, but is also knowledgeable about the trends affecting medical nutrition therapy practice. These advanced practice dietitians have developed expertise based on a broad and deep knowledge in medical nutrition therapy, pharmacology, pathophysiology, and co-morbidities of disease. They read, understand, and apply concepts from the research literature. They are also aware of their practice environment and take the initiative to shape that environment. They approach complex situations confidently, extracting and examining information from a wealth of sources and instantly presenting a solution tailored for the situation at hand.

Advanced practice dietitians may be found at work in the community, private practice, physician's offices, home care, long-term care, and acute care, or increasingly in a combination of these settings. These dietitians may consider themselves to be generalists or they may specialize in work with a particular patient population. These patients may be identified by age, disease, location, or use of a specific type of therapy. Advanced practice dietitians typically exercise a great deal of autonomy, making independent decisions, designing interventions, and prescribing and implementing therapy.

In addition, advanced practice dietitians possess a breadth and balance of perspective on clinical situations. They use scientific inquiry to discern the essential aspects of the situation at hand, and they easily and quickly integrate the plan for medical nutrition therapy into the most complex medical care. And they are generous: Advanced practice dietitians share their practice experience, educational background, and scientific approach with a wide network of colleagues. They are sought after as teachers by a variety of individuals and groups. Their knowledge of leadership and awareness of the practice context enable them to shape both their own practice and their professional environment. To do so, these healthcare professionals initiate and implement new policies, practices, and programs.

Advanced practice dietitians are thought leaders who initiate new approaches to issues. They create new information or look at existing information in new ways. Advanced practice dietitians lead change, continually moving themselves, their practice, and those around them forward. Although they have mastered the traditional rules and paradigms and the evidence supporting them, these dietitians have moved beyond a rule-bound approach. That is, they no longer need rules and paradigms to make decisions. Instead, they use their knowledge and practice experience to develop and initiate new practices and paradigms.

Rather than focus on absolute right or wrong, advanced practice dietitians are comfortable with ambiguity. These individuals critique—rather than criticize—their own practice and that of others. They apply judgment in their own practice, but are not judgmental of the practice of others. When asked a question, they often respond with a question, seeking clarity or more information before offering an answer. In keeping with the scientific tradition so important to dietitians, they confidently offer one of several correct answers, and can provide a clear rationale and quote supporting evidence for their choice. More often than not, however, the advanced practice dietitian is not asked for an explanation or rationale. Colleagues simply accept the proffered solution, knowing intuitively or by experience the rational thinking and scientific basis used to derive it.

Advanced medical nutrition therapy practitioners are recognized by others. Advanced practice dietitians are recognized by nurses, physicians, and other health professionals who comment on their contributions to patient care. In the words of one employer, "There is really something special about the way that dietitian adjusts the insulin and diet for diabetic patients. She just knows what to do." In the words of another, "She doesn't have to go to the literature—she knows the literature."

Although advanced practice dietitians are recognized for their expertise, they often find it difficult to define and describe their special skills. It is typical of experts, when asked about their thought processes, or how they know what they know, to respond with a remark such as "You wouldn't understand" or "It would take too long to explain."[1] Advanced practice dietitians will frequently state, "I can't explain what I do" or, as one advanced practice dietitian said, "I just use my sense of smell." These seemingly simple answers belie a wealth of knowledge and experience that is valuable to patients, employers, and other dietitians alike.

Advanced practice dietitians may also have difficulty in describing how they obtained their expertise. Many simply state that they have learned over time or that they have learned from experience. A few acknowledge mentors, and some mention formal education, including specific courses. Others point to scholarly activities, especially reading the literature or preparing presentations, as contributing to their expertise. Some dietitians make note of their interactions with practitioners from other disciplines as forming or shaping their expertise. Others mention acquiring knowledge outside dietetics as broadening their expertise.

Illuminating the expertise and the route to obtaining that expertise would serve as the basis for developing another level of dietetic practice. With a clear understanding of advanced practice expertise, the dietetics profession can educate, credential, and promote advanced practice. Thus the central purpose of this book is to explore advanced dietetics practice in medical nutrition therapy.

TRENDS AFFECTING THE NEED FOR ADVANCED PRACTICE DIETITIANS

Dietetics is part of a larger group of health professions that are, in turn, part of the healthcare industry. Thus the concepts of advanced practice and advanced practice dietitians themselves are subject to other trends within health care. For this reason, we next review several trends in health care and discuss how they might affect the advanced practice dietitian.

Continued Growth in Knowledge

There is an increasing awareness of the effects of food and nutrient intake on the health of the population. According to the Centers for Disease Control and Prevention (CDC), improper diet and exercise is the second most important preventable cause of disease after smoking.[2] A mounting body of evidence indicates that even small changes in nutrient intake may prevent disease and related comorbidities.[3–5] New findings in immunology and nutriogenomics inform therapies that maximize nutrition outcomes.[6,7] The expanding knowledge base means that dietitians are no longer limited to implementing a single intervention, but rather typically select from an array of diet and nutrition modifications and a variety of counseling techniques so as to meet the specific needs of particular patients. The variety and complexity of nutrient modifications are expected to increase even more in the future as genetic profiles become more available and dietitians use this information to design even more highly tailored disease prevention plans for individual patients.

At the same time that the amount of nutrition information available is increasing, knowledge in collateral areas is being recommended to increase practice effectiveness. For example, dietitians have been included in the Institute of Medicine's recommendations to implement new patient care models, to learn and use informatics, to participate as collaborators on interdisciplinary teams, to develop skills in evidence-based practice, and to improve quality of services provided.[8] In some practice settings, dietitians face complex legal and ethical challenges that require more than a cursory review of these topics. Legislative, economic, and regulatory issues have all dramatically affected the settings in which dietitians practice. Thus dietitians are challenged to develop not only skills in the scientific basis of practice, but also a breadth of practice-related knowledge and skills.

Some would disagree that topics such as genetics, informatics, the regulatory or legal basis of practice, or even analysis of the results of research studies in medical nutrition therapy should be considered "advanced." Others tend to label new information as "advanced" simply because it is new. Clearly, the unremitting flow of new knowledge and scientific information will prompt discussion and debate as to the depth and breadth of knowledge and skill needed for basic, specialist, or advanced practice. Individual dietitians will need to develop an appropriate depth and breadth of current and evolving knowledge and expertise to meet practice requirements for current and future practice roles. Advanced practice dietitians can participate in this debate and serve as a filter for new nutrition knowledge by selecting, evaluating, incorporating, and disseminating new knowledge and skills.

Continued Growth in Jobs

In 2006, the U.S. Bureau of Labor Statistics increased the predicted growth rate for jobs in dietetics. Based on its figures, new jobs for dietitians are expected to grow faster than average or between 18% and 26% through 2014.[9] The forecasted growth in clinical dietetics is consistent with increasing interest on the part of the general population in food and nutrient intake as a means to maintain health and prevent disease. It is also consistent with anticipated increases in chronic diseases such as obesity and diabetes and the aging of the U.S. population—both trends that will increase the need for nutrition services. Opportunities may also be created by predicted shortages of physicians in specialties such as endocrinology, nephrology, and critical care medicine, where nutrition is a major part of treatment.[10] All of these factors point to a wealth of opportunities for advanced practice dietitians.

Employers will determine whether they need dietitians with advanced practice skills to fill some of the new positions they are creating. Some would argue that cost pressures will work against an increased number of advanced practice dietetics. However, advanced practice dietitians who can document improved outcomes of their care will be in a position to demonstrate their value to employers, payers, and legislators. Recent data suggest that employers currently recognize and value advanced dietetics practice.[11] In the future, advanced practice dietitians will be needed to develop and fill new jobs, and to educate and train dietitians needed to fill the newly emerging jobs at all levels of practice.

Increasing Regulation

Health care is a high-risk industry and, therefore, is highly regulated. Concerns about safety in healthcare institutions will likely influence the trend toward increasing healthcare regulation.[12] In the United States, healthcare facilities must meet the Centers for Medicare and Medicaid Services' (CMS) Conditions for Participation by obtaining accreditation from the Joint Commission of the Healthcare Facilities Accreditation Program, a state's Department of Health, or other organizations.[13] The U.S. Department of Health and Human Services (DHHS) is responsible for administering privacy regulations in this country.[14] The practice of healthcare professionals is also regulated by complex credentialing and licensure systems. In some states, dietitians have a regulated Scope of Practice[15]; in other states, dietitians are subject to a Business and Professional Code. Advanced practice dietitians can become experts in how these regulations are developed and administered, and then influence these policies by moving into senior roles in organizations that develop and administer healthcare regulations.

Scientific and Economic Accountability

Traditional medical nutrition therapy has been pragmatically based, with dietitians adopting a "whatever works" approach. Today, this approach is no longer considered valid: Patients, employers, governments at all levels, and the insurance industry are demanding better value for their healthcare dollars.[16] As a result, new and existing medical nutrition therapies are being judged against rigorous scientific and economic standards.

The ability to analyze evidence documenting the results of nutrition intervention is an increasingly important skill. Advanced practice dietitians with expertise in evidence analysis are needed both to evaluate existing evidence and to design scientifically sound interventions. Those with expertise in measuring outcomes are needed to document effective and efficient medical nutrition therapies. In cases where there is no evidence, advanced practice dietitians are needed to develop and test new interventions, to select the most appropriate intervention that improves outcomes, and to reject traditional, comfortable or attractive, but unnecessary or ineffective practices. Advanced practice dietitians will be asked to analyze evidence and to develop guidelines that reflect not only sound science but also knowledge of the practice setting and the specific patient population. They can lead these efforts to demonstrate the scientific and economic value of medical nutrition therapy if they work with their colleagues to develop outcomes measurement and outcomes research skills.

Changes in Skills and Settings

Increasing workloads for all health professionals are the result of continued economic pressure on healthcare systems. As a result, some activities are being realigned. Tasks formerly performed exclusively by physicians have been shifted to other providers.[17] In some settings, dietitians are developing and implementing nontraditional skills willingly delegated by overworked physicians. In other settings, they are developing skills to fill a need or skills that complement nutrition interventions that fill a need in the practice setting. In all settings, there is less time available for training, so that dietitians are responsible for obtaining these skills on their own. In some settings, physicians or nutrition managers are not available to direct patient care, so that dietitians are responsible for independently implementing interventions and monitoring the results. In other settings, sophisticated patients or clients bring treatments or interventions that they wish to implement and seek advice from health professionals concerning their implementation or benefit. Advanced practice dietitians must have the maturity and confidence to function productively within this ever-changing environment.

Changes in Roles

On a daily basis, the media provide the public with an almost unlimited supply of enticing health and nutrition information. Both health professionals and their patients can access in-depth knowledge on these topics with just two or three clicks of a computer mouse. As a consequence, physicians and consumers alike have increasingly sophisticated knowledge of nutrition. Unfortunately, they are also susceptible to the proliferation of nutrition misinformation. Physicians and the patients they refer require a knowledgeable intermediary to help them sift through the available information and to develop an appropriate, evidence-based plan of nutritional care.

As health care changes, dietitians are practicing in a variety of locations, which are themselves changing. In some of these locations, advanced practice dietitians are sole practitioners autonomously managing a patient caseload. In other settings, advanced practice dietitians collaborate with members of an interdisciplinary team, performing interchangeable roles with physicians, pharmacists, and nurses to deliver comprehensive care. Advanced practice dietitians may develop protocols for disease state management or informatics organizations. They may also review nutrition data for policy makers or industry. In healthcare organizations, advanced practice dietitians initiate and manage clinical programs and serve as clinical researchers. They are leading their practice into new areas by creating new products, services, interventions, protocols, and roles.

Increasing Educational Requirements

Today, entry-level education standards are increasing across all health professions in the United States.[18] For example, the physical therapy and pharmacy professions now require a first professional or doctoral degree for entry-level preparation.[19,20] Thus all new pharmacists and physical therapists are educated similarly to physicians and dentists—that is, at the doctoral level. Similarly, the audiology and occupational therapy professions no longer accept baccalaureate degrees as preparation for entry-level practice: The occupational therapy profession mandates a master's degree for entry-level practice, and audiology is moving toward doctoral preparation for entry-level practice.[21,22] The nursing profession has recommended a requirement of a practice doctorate degree for nurse practitioners, clinical nurse specialists, certified registered nurse anesthetists, and nurse midwives.[23]

The rationale for this trend includes the need for increased time to learn the skills expected by today's patients and employers, employer expectations for a more confident entry-level practitioner, increasing knowledge requirements for entry-level practice, and the increased possibility of Medicare reimbursement for services provided by independent or mid-level practitioners educated at the doctoral level. The role of economic motives in these salary decisions is unstated, but salary increases have accrued to members of these professions as they increase their educational requirements. In the future, advanced practice dietitians will need similar education to other health professionals if they hope to obtain similar salary and reimbursement benefits.

THE RATIONALE FOR ADVANCED MEDICAL NUTRITION THERAPY PRACTICE

In discussing professional roles and responsibilities, some dietitians and employers have asked whether advanced practice dietitians are truly needed. In addition, dietitians and their employers have questioned whether the healthcare system has enough resources to support additional levels of practice. Educators are also concerned about how advanced practice dietitians will be educated and trained. They cite a lack of resources, including a shortage of trained faculty to support advanced practice dietetics education programs. Some educators insist that dietitians receive sufficient education at the baccalaureate level and see no reason to upgrade the knowledge and skills taught to dietitians.

At the same time, today's dietitians are developing and moving into roles and responsibilities that would have been unthinkable 15 years ago. A recent survey documented both that positions are available for advanced practice dietitians and that dietitians are interested in advanced practice education.[11] Clinical nutrition managers are developing career ladders to reward and retain dietitians who develop advanced practice skills. At least one education program for advanced practice dietitians exists.[24] The Commission on Dietetic Registration includes advanced practice concepts in its practice audits and conducted a separate audit of advanced practice in 2007. The Standards of Dietetic Practice identify three levels of professional practice: generalist, specialist, and advanced practice.[25]

Key structures supporting advanced practice are evolving such that the dietetics profession is clearly moving toward incorporating a higher level of practice. The specific benefits of advanced practice in dietetics to patients, practitioners, employers, the profession, and the healthcare industry are outlined in the following sections.

Value of Advanced Practice to Patients

Advanced practice dietitians provide value to their patients by integrating a greater breadth and depth of knowledge into practice. They use these extra skills to improve nutrition outcomes for individual patients, groups, and populations. Advanced practice dietitians incorporate research-based, advanced-level information about nutrition pharmacology, nutrition pathophysiology, disease co-morbidities, and medical nutrition therapy into practice. They will have graduate-level preparation and extensive experience with different counseling theories and other sophisticated nutrition interventions. The advanced level practitioner will use these skills to resolve complex nutrition diagnoses by skillfully organizing and implementing multiple interventions.

Value of Advanced Practice to Dietitians

Advanced dietetic practice is of value to dietitians who wish to advance their careers. A clearly defined path to advanced practice, including both the education and credentials necessary to reach the next step on the career ladder, can be used for career planning purposes and to facilitate upward mobility within the profession. Advanced practice is anticipated to increase job satisfaction for those dietitians whose career aspirations include more autonomous positions. A formal system of advanced practice should provide dietitians with the confidence, maturity, and clinical skills to meet the demands of new practice settings and to create new practice roles.

Value of Advanced Practice to Employers

Advanced practice dietitians can benefit employers by providing high-quality care and documenting outcomes. They can develop strategic initiatives and support them by developing new products or programs that result in increased referrals and justification for expanded services. In turn, incorporation of advanced practice roles within organizations will allow employers to develop career ladders. Organizations that successfully mentor basic or specialist level staff to a higher level of practice may, in turn, reduce their expenses associated with employee turnover. A clear differentiation of skill levels will aid in matching the skill levels of dietitians with the skills needed for specific positions.

Value of Advanced Practice to the Profession

Many medical nutrition therapy advances of the last two decades have been based on work done by physician or basic science researchers. Although this approach generates valuable information, physicians and basic scientists typically have little interest in answering research questions specific to dietetics practice. While dietitians have incorporated their findings into practice, dozens of questions have not yet been answered by these groups or individuals. Thus opportunities exist for advanced practice dietitians with practice-based research skills to collaborate with basic and applied scientists to develop and investigate questions specific to dietetics practice.

An unknown number of dietitians leave practice and enter other fields. Some educators take pride in the decision of their graduates to leave dietetics for careers as physicians, physician assistants, or nurses. Overall, however, this trend is detrimental to the profession. When tenured advanced practitioners exit the profession, they take with them accumulated knowledge and experience that can create a void of professional expertise. This knowledge must then be recreated by others, who in turn are ultimately lured to other professions that offer greater opportunities. Clearly, creation of a system that educates, trains, and credentials advanced practice dietitians could not only help to retain practitioners, but also ensure that they use their expertise to advance the profession.

Value of Advanced Practice to the Healthcare System

Further stratification of the profession may help meet the demand to deliver the right care, in the right location, to the right people, at the right time, and at the right price.[16] Advanced practice dietitians can discern which care is appropriate for which patients, design systems to identify those patients who will benefit from nutrition intervention, develop those interventions, and apply them in a manner that matches intervention with need and reduces ineffective or unnecessary care. The greater benefit to the healthcare system, however, is the application of the accumulated knowledge and expertise of advanced practice to nutrition diagnosis. Over time, advanced practice dietitians could make significant inroads into improving improper diet, the second most preventable cause of disease.[2]

SUMMARY

In most health professions, there is a clear progression from beginning practitioner to seasoned expert. While such a progression may exist in dietetics, it is not clearly articulated.

Advanced dietetics practice exists, but a clearer vision is needed to design the supporting structures: a defined educational pathway with appropriate coursework and practice experiences, a credentialing mechanism that certifies expertise, and a well-defined set of skills that have value in the marketplace. The following chapters in this text will define and describe the knowledge, skills, education, and training of the advanced practice dietitian.

KEY POINTS

- Opportunities for dietitians at all levels of practice—basic, specialty, and generalist—are expected to increase as new jobs in dietetics are created at an above-average rate.
- Trends in health care, including growth of knowledge, jobs, regulations and accountability, and changes in roles and practice settings, favor the continued development of advanced practice in medical nutrition therapy.
- Advanced practice in dietetics is expected to bring value to patients, to dietitians, to their employers, to the profession, and to the healthcare system as a whole.

REFERENCES

1. Schon DA. *The reflective practitioner.* New York, NY: Basic Books, 1983.
2. Mokdad AH, Marks JS, Stroup DF, Gerberding JL. Actual causes of death in the United States. *Journal of the American Medical Association* 2004;291(10):1238–1245.
3. Appel LJ, Brands MW, Daniels SR, Karanja N, Elmer PJ, Sacks FM. Dietary approaches to prevent and treat hypertension: A scientific statement from the American Heart Association. *Hypertension* 2006;47(2):296–308.
4. Holmes A, Sanderson B, Maisiak R, Brown A, Bittner V. Dietitian services are associated with improved patient outcomes and the MEDFICTS dietary assessment questionnaire is a suitable outcome measure in cardiac rehabilitation. *Journal of the American Dietetic Association* 2005;105(10):1533–1540.
5. McGeehee MM, Johnson EQ, Rasmussen HM, Sahyoun N, Lynch MM, Carey M. Benefits and cost of medical nutrition therapy by registered dietitians for patients with hypercholesterolemia. *Journal of the American Dietetic Association* 1995;95(9):1041–1043.
6. Debusk R, Fogarty C, Ordovas J, Kornman K. Nutritional genomics in practice: Where do we begin? *Journal of the American Dietetic Association* 2005;105(4):589–598.
7. German J, Watkins S, Fay L. Metabolomics in practice: Emerging knowledge to guide future dietetic advice toward individualized health. *Journal of the American Dietetic Association* 2005;105(9):1425–1432.
8. *Health professions education: A bridge to quality.* Washington, DC: Institute of Medicine, 2003.
9. U.S. Department of Labor: Bureau of Labor Statistics. Health diagnosing and treating practitioners. Available at http://www.bls.gov/oco/ocos077.htm. Accessed January 6, 2007.
10. Salesberg E, Grover A. Physician workforce shortages: Implications and issues for academic health centers and policymakers. *Academic Medicine* 2006;81(9):782–787.
11. Skipper A, Lewis NM. Clinical dietitians, employers, and educators are interested in advanced practice education and professional doctorate degrees in clinical nutrition. *Journal of the American Dietetic Association* 2006;106(12):2062–2066.
12. Kohn LT, Corrigan JM, Donaldson MS (eds.). *To err is human: Building a safer health system.* Washington, DC: Institute of Medicine, 2000.
13. Sprague L. *Hospital oversight in Medicare: Accreditation and deeming authority.* Washington, DC: George Washington University, 2005, p. 802.
14. National standards to protect the privacy of personal health information. Available at http://www.hhs.gov/ocr/hipaa/. Accessed January 9, 2007.
15. State licensure information. Available at: http://www.cdrnet.org/certifications/index.htm. Accessed January 1, 2007.
16. Institute of Medicine. *Crossing the quality chasm: A new health system for the 21st century.* Washington, DC: Institute of Medicine, 2001.
17. Druss BG, Marcus SC, Olfson M, Tanielian T, Pincus HA. Trends in care by nonphysician clinicians in the United States. *New England Journal of Medicine* 2003;348(2):130–137.
18. Skipper A, Lewis NM. A look at the educational preparation of the health diagnosing and treating professions: Do dietitians measure up? *Journal of the American Dietetic Association* 2005;105(3):420–427.

19. American Council on Pharmaceutical Education. Implementation procedures for accreditation standards and guidelines for the professional program in pharmacy leading to the doctor of pharmacy degree. Available at www.acpe-accredit.org/docs/pubs. Accessed July 20, 2003.

20. American Physical Therapy Association. Doctor of Physical Therapy (DPT) degree frequently asked questions. Available at http://www.apta.org. Accessed June 29, 2006.

21. Nodar RH. New audiology certification standards: What they mean to you. *ASHA* 1999;41(3):8.

22. American Occupational Therapy Association. Frequently asked questions regarding occupational therapy education. Available at http://www.aota.org/nonmembers/area2/links/links/link01.asp. Accessed June 22, 2006.

23. American Association of Colleges of Nursing. The essentials of doctoral education for advanced nursing practice. Available at http://www.aacn.nche.edu/DNP/pdf/Essentials.pdf. Accessed July 24, 2007.

24. Touger-Decker R. Advanced practice doctorate in clinical nutrition. *Topics in Clinical Nutrition* 2005;20(1):48–53.

25. Kieselhorst K, Skates J, Pritchett E. American Dietetic Association: Standards of practice in nutrition care and updated standards of professional performance. *Journal of the American Dietetic Association* 2005;105(4):614–645 (645.e611–645.e610).

A Historical and Contextual Perspective on Advanced Medical Nutrition Therapy

"Never measure the height of a mountain until you have reached the top. Then you will see how low it was." —Dag Hammersckjöld

The word "advanced" has been defined as "being beyond others in progress or ideas, being beyond the elementary or introductory, or as greatly developed beyond an initial stage."[1] In the professions, advanced level practitioners have expertise, defined as having, involving, or displaying special skill or knowledge derived from training or experience.[1] If these definitions are applied, advanced practice may be described as the application of special skills, knowledge, or expertise that is greatly developed beyond an initial stage.

There is a large body of knowledge about the acquisition and application of expertise in a wide variety of professions.[2] A review of various models of expert or advanced practice is useful to better understand what expertise is and how it develops. It is also useful to understand how various models of expertise have been applied in dietetics. The first section of this chapter describes several models of advanced practice skills and expertise derived from research in a variety of professions. The second portion of the chapter contains more specific information relating to advanced practice in health care. The final part of the chapter offers a brief history of advanced practice in dietetics.

ADVANCED PRACTICE MODELS

The models that follow represent several major trends in thinking about the nature of advanced practice and the way in which expertise develops. These models are based on conversations between the author and leaders in dietetics from the 1989 role delineation studies, through the time of the 2007 advanced practice audit. Where possible, the reader is referred to supporting literature. However, this section is intended to stimulate thinking rather than to provide an exhaustive review of the literature on the topic of expertise.

The Naturalistic or Unschooled Genius Model

In this model, advanced practitioners or experts appear spontaneously without specific education, training, or experience. Proponents of this model advocate that qualities needed for expertise, such as intellect and motivation, are innate and cannot be developed by education, practice, or experience. The naturalistic model purports that individuals simply begin to function at a very high level early in a star-studded career. Examples of the "unschooled genius" performing at a level far beyond what he or she has been taught include the musicians Amadeus Mozart and Louis Armstrong, the inventor Thomas Edison, and the politicians Benjamin Franklin and Harry Truman. These examples, along with ones from dietetics, are inevitably presented by those opposed to formalizing educational or credentialing requirements for advanced level practitioners.

The naturalistic model has its roots in the work of Sir Frances Galton, whose *Hereditary Genius* was published in 1869.[3] This model is no longer widely accepted, however. In an extensive review of the subsequent literature, Ericsson et al. convincingly refuted the notion of naturally occurring expertise.[4] Based on their own extensive research and that of others, Ericsson et al. established that innate characteristics play a minimal role in the development of expertise. To support this conclusion, these authors cited dozens of studies in domains as diverse as music, typing, mathematics, and athletic performance showing the positive effects of deliberative practice in improving even very high-level performance.[4]

The individual accomplishments of dietitians who were undereducated for advanced practice roles are difficult to deny, and anecdotal records of self-taught expertise will always exist. With careful planning and disciplined, individual study, dietitians may be able to acquire the complex skills needed by advanced practice dietitians. Nevertheless, self-directed learning is likely to be inefficient when compared to a formal curriculum of study and mentored practice experience. Waiting for expert, advanced practice dietitians to appear spontaneously seems unlikely to produce sufficient numbers of consistently trained advanced practice dietitians to meet future practice needs. An additional concern with the naturalistic model is that it is inconsistent with a compensation and reimbursement system based on education and credentials.

The Longevity Model

The longevity approach presumes that skills increase with increased experience and that advanced practice automatically appears as practice experience accumulates. This model has its roots in the guild system devised in the Middle Ages. It has been used extensively in skilled trades. In some civil service positions, longevity figures heavily into wages and benefits. It would be difficult to justify advanced practice based on longevity alone, but research supports the concept of longevity as a prerequisite to expertise. In several professions, studies show that it takes 10 or more years to acquire mastery or expertise in performing complex tasks.[4] In fact, this finding is prevalent across enough fields that it has been dubbed the "10-year rule."[2] In dietetics, this model is somewhat supported by the work of Bradley et al., who identified a different and more advanced skill set that appeared when practitioners acquired seven to eight years of experience.[5]

The longevity model is attractive because of its simplicity. In reality, it may be too simple. In professions where expertise has been studied, fewer than 10% of professionals practice at an advanced level. In dietetics, authors of the single contemporary study on the topic of longevity estimated that 8.9% of the dietitians sampled practiced at an advanced level.[5] If one accepts these findings, then it seems clear that only a relatively small proportion of the profession practices at an advanced level. If most professionals enter practice at about age 25, retire at about age 65, and are evenly distributed by age, then as many as 50% to 75% of professionals would have more than 10 years of experience. In dietetics, the small proportion of experienced dietitians meeting advanced practice criteria (8.9%), compared to the larger number of practitioners with more than 10 years of experience (50% to 75%), suggests that there are more determinants of advanced level practice than longevity alone.[5]

The Expertise Continuum Model

Current thinking about advanced practice can be traced to Dreyfus and Dreyfus.[6] These brothers, a decision scientist and a philosopher, worked at RAND Corporation during the 1960s as part of a group studying artificial intelligence. They sought first to understand the complex thinking used to play chess or fly airplanes and then to program that thinking into computers. One result of their research was a scheme to differentiate skill levels along a continuum of expertise. The five levels of skills the Dreyfus brothers identified were novice, advanced beginner, competence, proficiency, and expertise.

In addition to identifying levels of expertise, in *Mind Over Machine*, Dreyfus and Dreyfus described expert performance. This description is helpful as we consider how a dietitian performs expertly. Dreyfus and Dreyfus described expertise as experiencing an act rather than consciously performing a set of tasks.[6] They cited the example of driving a car, in which the expert experiences driving, rather than consciously turning, speeding, or slowing the car. Dreyfus and Dreyfus further describe expert performance as "seeing" the situation and solutions based on similar patterns that trigger a response.[6]

In *Blink*, Gladwell presented a striking example of expertise.[7] He recounted the story of an authority on Greek art who was invited to preview a statue under consideration for purchase by a noted museum. The curator unveiled the statue and quickly said, "It isn't ours yet, but it will be." The expert instantly replied, "I'm sorry to hear that," recognizing the statue as a fake within one or two seconds and before even examining it.[7] In this situation, the expert did not stop to reflect on her own experience or carefully calculate the options, but rather proceeded instinctively based on extensive expertise. When asked how she knew the statue was a fake, she could not explain. In another incident, Gladwell relayed the story of a world-class tennis player who observed other players and predicted a double fault as often as 17 of 18 times. Interestingly, the tennis player was unable to describe exactly how he knew that a player would double fault.

These scenarios provided by Dreyfus and Dreyfus and by Gladwell are quickly understood by advanced practice dietitians. They use a very similar process to hone questions that will enable them to obtain the two or three crucial pieces of information needed to differentiate between two complex nutrition diagnoses, but are unable to explain how they knew which two pieces of information were needed.

The Practitioner Characteristics Model

This model is based on individual practitioner characteristics such as educational qualifications, years of experience, leadership activities, specialty certifications, and practice areas. For example, Bradley et al. described advanced practice dietitians as having a master's degree; a minimum of eight years experience; multiple professional role positions with complex and diverse responsibilities and functions; a diverse network of broad, geographically dispersed professional contacts; and an innovative, creative, and intuitive approach to practice that reflects a global perspective.[5] Practitioner characteristics are popular measures of advanced practice and figure prominently in career laddering schemes because they are objective and easily measured.

The practitioner characteristics model is prone to the same problematic issue as the longevity model—namely, it is possible that all practitioners described by a given set of characteristics will not practice at an advanced level. Some critics of this model condemn practitioner characteristics such as elected offices or leadership in volunteer organizations as being a popularity contest rather than a true measure of practice expertise. Practitioner characteristic models are also objectionable to compensation specialists who prefer to focus on productivity, outcomes, or licensure requirements to justify positions and salaries.

Another problem with practitioner characteristic models that incorporate a master's degree is the limited number of master's degrees that are specifically designed to improve medical nutrition therapy skills. Many dietitians obtain master's degrees in nutrition science or nutritional biochemistry, through programs that are designed to prepare students for research rather than practice. It is unknown whether these degrees improve medical nutrition therapy skills. It is also unknown if the dietitians in Bradley et al.'s sample held master's degrees in areas related to dietetics or if they were in other fields.

The Task Hierarchy Model

Perhaps the most widely used model applied specifically to advanced dietetics practice is the hierarchical model of tasks created in the late 1970s by dietitians working in foodservice management practice.[8] This task hierarchy presumed that management functions were performed at different levels by people with different levels of expertise based on the authority that accompanied their work position. The terms "no involvement," "doing," "supervising," and "setting policy" were used to represent a continuum of practice, where "doing" was the lowest level and "setting policy" was the highest level.

The dietetics profession has completed several carefully conducted attempts to delineate advanced practice roles using variations on the task hierarchy models.[9–12] Based on the results of these studies, there is a perception that advanced practice dietitians function primarily in management roles. This conclusion is not surprising if the verbs applied to the tasks studies are examined carefully. Of the four levels, "doing" applies to the practice of medical nutrition therapy, whereas "supervising" and "setting policy" denote management roles. Absence of a second or third level that distinguishes actually "doing" or "performing" tasks limits advanced practice to those who are promoted to a management position. Thus the language used by these investigators was not designed to detect expert or advanced clinical practice, but rather to identify promotion to a supervisory or managerial level.

The task hierarchy model reflects a problem in accurately describing advanced practice activities. When asked about their clinical responsibilities, dietitians typically respond, "I do the pediatric floor," "I work with transplant patients," or "I'm in long-term care." That is, dietitians describe practice in terms of the patients treated or the setting where care is delivered. This vocabulary is not rich enough to convey their level of involvement in nutrition diagnosis or intervention. Thus the focus is on the patient population served (i.e., what the dietitian "knows") rather than the level of practice (i.e., what the dietitian "does").

Difficulty in describing advanced practice might arise from the limitations imposed by an insufficient vocabulary, or it might arise from the inability to put into words what is done instinctively. Dreyfus and Dreyfus related an anecdote in which a nurse tried to explain psychosis, a disease she knew inside out, to novice nurses. She stated, "All I am really trying to do is find words within the jargon to talk about something that I don't think is particularly describable."[6] The difficulty of describing advanced practice dietetics is similar to the difficulty an experienced driver would have in explaining how to drive to someone who had never seen a car. The expert driver experiences the act of driving, while the novice driver consciously reviews a specific set of actions needed to set the car in motion. Similarly, an advanced practice dietitian finds it equally difficult to describe how to distinguish between nutritional or non-nutritional causes of failure to thrive in an infant to a hospital administrator and a team of consultants visiting a pediatric clinic.

The Marketable Skills Model

In the marketable skills model, the dietitian acquires advanced skills that generate revenue or reduce costs for patients, employers, or payers. The marketplace determines success based on economic terms. Many dietitians receive a salary, but others bill for their services and are paid on a per-case basis. Under the marketable skills model, success is measured in monetary terms. Dietitians are more successful if they are more efficient or work more hours. They are also more successful if they treat grateful patients who refer their friends and family members for care.

Dietitians who maintain a good reputation in the community ensure continued referrals and a constant income stream.

The healthcare market values services according to a hierarchy of knowledge, skills, and risk. Healthcare professionals are required to have knowledge for entry-level credentialing and are expected to maintain current knowledge of practice. They are also expected to be skillful in using the knowledge they possess, which is the reason for supervised practice, residency, or fellowship training. In addition, healthcare professionals are expected to assume risk, which is defined as "active intervention with the potential for medical compromise."[1] The healthcare marketplace has typically bestowed the greatest rewards on those who apply a great deal of knowledge and skill to perform high-risk interventions that result in improved outcomes.

The mean salaries for clinical nurse specialists, nurse practitioners, and nurse anesthetists provide a clear example of how the market rewards advanced practice nurses according to the mix of knowledge, skills, and risk that they apply in practice. All three groups of nurses obtain a master of science degree in nursing (M.S.N.) followed by supervised clinical experience, but each group functions differently in the work setting. Clinical nurse specialists have an extensive depth of knowledge that enables them to serve as content experts—for example, training new nurses, advising experienced nurses on new developments in the field, and developing policies and procedures. Nurse practitioners are much more "hands-on," diagnosing and treating disease and prescribing medications for patients with common medical problems. Nurse anesthetists provide high-risk medications in the form of anesthesia. According to data from the National Nurses Survey, clinical nurse specialists earn a mean of $52,383, while the mean salary for nurse practitioners ($64,538) is 23% higher; the mean salary for nurse anesthetists ($93,787) is 79% higher than for clinical specialists and 45% higher than for nurse practitioners.[13] This example clearly demonstrates that the marketplace rewards higher-risk activities.

Many dietitians have taken advantage of opportunities to be trained in marketable, nontraditional, but dietetics-related skills. For example, dietitians in critical care have developed skills in performing abdominal exams and placing small bowel feeding tubes so as to facilitate enteral feeding.[14,15] Dietitians in long-term care perform oral examinations and dysphagia screening.[16] There are reports of dietitians in home care who draw blood, take vital signs, and change dressings. Renal dietitians adjust phosphate binders and iron supplements and order recirculation studies. Dietitians working with patients who have diabetes adjust insulin doses and schedules and perform nerve conduction studies. In some institutions, dietitians have obtained clinical privileges that permit them to order high-risk medications such as parenteral nutrition.[17–19] In other institutions, dietitians order vitamins, modified diets, enteral feedings, and biochemical tests.[20,21]

Marketable skills for dietitians are many and varied, and not all are advanced. Some skills, such as drawing blood and taking vital signs, are taught to patient care technicians in a few hours. Others, such as feeding tube placement, are more time-consuming to learn and engender greater risk.[22] In some cases, it is clear that skills enhance efficiency, reduce costs, or increase referrals, and dietitians have negotiated higher salaries for performing them. In other cases, dietitians have been content with the increased job satisfaction or more efficient practice that resulted from learning advanced skills. While not all dietitians will negotiate extra compensation for adding more skills to their repertoire, it is clear that the new skills must be of value in the marketplace to result in additional compensation.

Institution-Specific Models

A recent trend in dietetics is to stratify practice based on a model approved and implemented within a single institution. These models may include various policies, procedures, standards, algorithms, preapproved protocols, and clinical ladders that define advanced practice within a single institution. Such models have evolved based on unique situations within institutions, and consequently they vary according to resource availability and sometimes even the personalities of the individuals involved. Some of these models constitute advanced practice; others emphasize longevity, productivity, or tradition.

The accomplishments of individuals who have developed institution-specific advanced practice models should be both recognized and commended. These models reflect the collective effort of many dietitians who wish to elevate practice. Nevertheless, an autonomous profession should not delegate the authority to regulate itself to employers. The dietetics profession cannot rely on thousands of institutions to consistently and fairly specify the qualifications of advanced level practitioners. Delegating the authority of the profession to regulate itself to employers will result in confusion, inconsistent practice, and a fragmented standard of care. Profession-wide criteria, agreed upon and promoted by a national organization, are needed as the basis for uniform education, practice, and reimbursement for services.

Advanced Practice Models: A Summary

The models presented here reflect several differing viewpoints advocated by dietitians who seek to promote advanced practice. It is unknown whether any of these models might be applied without modification to the dietetics profession. They do serve to focus attention on the major schools of thought in the area of advanced practice, however, and they provide a framework for further discussion and debate.

THE HEALTHCARE CONTEXT

Health care is a large industry representing a substantial portion of the U.S. economy. It is the primary employer for dozens of healthcare professions, including medicine, nursing, pharmacy, physical therapy, and dietetics. Dietitians wishing to establish advanced practice will need to be aware of the established education, credentials, and laws and regulations governing advanced practice so that their preparation and practice will be consistent with industry expectations. This section provides a brief overview of some key advanced practice concepts already in place within the industry.

Routes to Expertise

Advanced practice or expertise is typically established following lengthy and rigorous educational preparation. For example, physicians complete medical school, residency, and fellowships before entering practice.[23] This process may take as long as 10 years. Physicians do not appear to have a formal advanced practice structure in place. Instead, they depend on specialty training in areas such as pediatrics, psychiatry, obstetrics and gynecology, medicine, or surgery. They follow that with sub-specialty fellowships in areas such as gastroenterology, infectious disease, or nephrology and then become board certified in those sub-specialties. In recent years, this model has been adopted by the pharmacy and physical therapy professions as well.[24]

Nurses achieve advanced practice status following completion of an advanced degree in nursing, which is typically preceded by two years of practice experience and includes several months of supervised advanced practice.[25] Thus six to seven years of education and experience is required to become an advanced practice nurse. The nursing model allows for specialties within advanced practice. Advanced practice nurses obtain an M.S.N. and then engage in supervised clinical experience. On completion of the prerequisites, nurses are certified by examination in a particular area of practice, such as acute care, mental health, or pediatrics. Table 2–1 compares the definition and domains of advanced practice nursing to those for dietetics.[26]

Table 2-1 Definitions and Core Competencies for Advanced Practice Nurses and Dietitians

Advanced Practice Nursing	Advanced Practice Dietetics
Definition[26]	**Definition**[27]
"Manifests a high level of expertise in the assessment, diagnosis, and treatment of complex responses of individuals, families, or communities to actual or potential health problems, prevention of illness and injury, maintenance of wellness, and provision of comfort"	"An RD who has acquired the expert knowledgebase, complex decision-making skills, and clinical competencies for expanded practice, the characteristics of which are shaped by the context in which the RD practices"
Primary Criteria[28]	**Practitioner Characteristics**[29]
Graduate education	Master's degree
Certification	Professional role positions
Practice focused on patient/family	Experience
	Approach to practice
	Professional role contacts
	Professional achievement
Core Competencies[28]	**Core Competencies**
Direct practice	None
Expert coaching and guidance	
Consultation	
Research skills	
Clinical and professional leadership	
Collaboration	
Ethical decision-making skills	

It is interesting to note that the degrees used by these health professions are professional degrees. For example, physicians obtain a doctor of medicine degree (M.D.), pharmacists obtain a doctor of pharmacy degree (Pharm.D.), and nurses obtain an M.S.N., which may soon become a doctorate in nursing practice. These degrees require a baccalaureate degree as a prerequisite, and courses result in an advanced degree. However, the courses that serve as the basis for advanced practice are followed by or integrated with supervised professional practice. As a result, these degree programs are not open to students from other fields; they are profession specific, designed to educate a single type of health professional for professional practice.

The pharmacy and physical therapy professions have patterned the recent changes undertaken in their education and training programs on the physician model for education. Both professions now use the doctoral degree as a prerequisite to practice. They provide extensive education and training prior to credentialing, and offer specialty training in the form of residencies and fellowships.

Figure 2–1 provides more detail on the education, training, and market value for selected health diagnosing and treating professionals. It suggests that more education correlates with higher salaries except in the case of nursing, where well-publicized shortages have been used to justify salary increases.

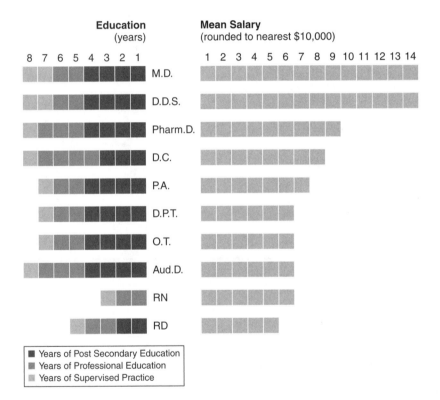

FIGURE 2–1 Educational Preparation and Mean Salary for Selected Health Diagnosing and Treating Professions

M.D. = Medical Doctor; D.D.S. = Doctor of Dental Surgery; Pharm.D. = Doctor of Pharmacy; D.C. = Doctor of Chiropractic; P.A. = Physician Assistant; D.P.T. = Doctor of Physical Therapy; O.T. = Occupational Therapist; Aud.D. = Doctor of Audiology; RN = Registered Nurse; RD = Registered Dietitian.

Bureau of Labor Statistics. May 2005 salary data. Available at http://www.bls.gov/oco/ocos077.htm. Accessed January 6, 2007.

Credentials

Examinations are typically used to document expertise and advanced practitioner status. For example, a nurse may complete a nurse practitioner, clinical nurse specialist, certified registered nurse anesthetist, or nurse midwife program. To work as a nurse practitioner, however, the nurse must also pass an exam in a specific area of practice, such as acute care, pediatrics, or adult mental health. Depending on the state licensing rules, the advanced practice nurse is also required to obtain a certain amount of continuing education annually. Physicians, pharmacists, and physical therapists are similarly licensed following examination and may also have to meet continuing education requirements to maintain licensure to practice. Within each state, licensure laws specify a scope of practice that defines the activities that advanced practice nurses, physicians, pharmacists, and others can perform.

Practice Autonomy

Within healthcare professions, the value of basic, specialty, and advanced practice is measured by practice autonomy. At least five criteria may be used to measure autonomy:

- Doctoral-level professional education
- The ability to diagnose and treat a specified set of diseases or conditions
- The ability to prescribe treatments, including drugs
- The level of independence in implementing interventions
- Direct reimbursement for services rendered

The highest level of autonomy is independent practitioner status. Independent practitioners include physicians, dentists, veterinarians, and podiatrists. Members of these professions have doctoral-level education, diagnose diseases and conditions according to specific criteria, prescribe medications, and perform medical and surgical treatments. These professionals may be paid directly for services rendered or their fees may be covered by various forms of insurance. They are subject to licensure laws and must obtain privileges to practice in hospitals that receive funding from the Centers for Medicare and Medicaid Services (CMS).[30] Once these criteria are met, however, these individuals practice independently, without oversight by another profession.

In the traditional system of authority and responsibility in health care, independent practitioners—primarily physicians—direct the activities of dependent practitioners, who include dietitians, nurses, pharmacists, physical therapists, medical technologists, and others. Direction from physicians takes the form of "orders" used to coordinate the activities of various caregivers while the physician was not present. It has become the norm that dependent practitioners deliver care only as ordered by an independent practitioner. Dependent practitioners have associate or baccalaureate degrees. They do not typically bill or receive payment directly for services rendered, but instead receive a salary from an employer who may bill for their services.

This traditional system is changing rapidly for several reasons. As health care has become more complex and expensive, delegation of tasks to the lowest-level person available has become the norm. Physicians can no longer afford to learn and perform all of the complex treatments needed by their patients. In response, other health professions have increased their skills and knowledge so as to fill these voids. As health care has moved farther from the hospital, physician oversight of skilled professionals by "ordering" care has become increasingly less practical.

As a result of these trends, a third level of practice has emerged. These non-physicians have prescriptive authority for drugs and treatments,[31] and they assume some of the responsibilities of a physician. They function with indirect physician oversight in the form of a collaborative practice agreement. These so-called mid-level practitioners include certified registered nurse anesthetists, nurse practitioners, nurse midwives, clinical nurse specialists, physician assistants, and, in some states, pharmacists. Mid-level practitioners are required to obtain rigorous, graduate-level education; to pass extra credentialing examinations; and to demonstrate physician supervision before being allowed to practice. The designation of mid-level practitioner is extended by the U.S. Drug Enforcement Administration (DEA) after state licensure laws are changed to accommodate prescriptive authority. The DEA maintains a list of drug prescribing privileges for practitioners in every state on its website.[22]

Reimbursement differs by profession for mid-level practitioners. Generally, advanced practice nurses are directly reimbursed for services performed, albeit at a lower rate than what a physician would receive for the same service. Pharmacy services have typically been covered as part of the overhead charged against drug revenues, so pharmacists rarely receive direct reimbursement for their services. Reimbursement is a major issue for physical therapists who are directly reimbursed for services performed. Currently, physical therapists are lobbying Congress in favor of legislation guaranteeing the right of patients to access physical therapy services directly, without physician referral. When passed, these laws will have the effect of making physical therapists independent practitioners.

The Healthcare Context: A Summary

Advanced practice models and a hierarchy of autonomy already exist within the healthcare industry. Advanced education and training, most often at the doctoral level, is a prerequisite for advanced practice. Advanced practice is well defined and clearly understood within the professions, and its definition has been codified into law in most states. Dietitians who wish to be recognized as advanced practitioners need to develop an understanding of how advanced practice skills are viewed within the healthcare industry so that they can establish their credibility as advanced level practitioners.

A BRIEF HISTORY OF ADVANCED PRACTICE IN DIETETICS

The dietetics profession was formed in Cleveland, Ohio, in 1917 by dietitians who met to discuss pressing food supply issues precipitated by World War I.[32] At the beginning, dietitians were focused on preparation of adequate, safe, nutritious food for large groups of individuals.[33] With the discoveries in nutrition during the 1920s through the 1950s, interest in therapeutic diets expanded, and by 1947 the majority of dietitians worked in clinical settings.[34] In 1955, dietetics adopted the philosophies of the American Hospital Association (AHA) and began to advance as a clinically focused profession.[34] By 1972, 70% of dietitians were employed in hospitals.[35] When interest in hospital malnutrition gained momentum in the late 1970s, an increasing need for therapeutic or clinical dietitians was recognized.[36,37] As knowledge of the role of diet in disease prevention and treatment accumulated, the need for clinical dietitians has continued to increase. Thus the number of clinical dietitians has grown rapidly over the last 30 years.

Dietetics has evolved to meet the generally accepted criteria for a profession as shown in Table 2–2. In 2003, The Institute of Medicine listed dietetics as one of the 10 largest and best-known health professions.[38] It is estimated that more than 60% of dietitians (approximately 45,000 professionals) now deliver direct clinical services to patients or clients in healthcare institutions and the community.[1] According to the 2005 Dietetic Practice Audit, approximately 75% of entry-level dietitians provide clinical services directly to patients.[12] The Bureau of Labor lists dietetics as one of 17 health diagnosing and treating occupations.[39]

The dietetics profession has defined dietetics as "the integration and application of principles derived from the sciences of food, nutrition, management,

Table 2–2 Characteristics of a Profession and Characteristics of the Dietetics Profession

Characteristics of a Profession	Characteristics of the Dietetics Profession	Examples
Code of ethics	The profession has developed and dietitians follow a code of ethics for practice	Code of Ethics for the Profession of Dietetics
Body of knowledge	The profession possesses a unique theoretical body of knowledge and science-based knowledge that leads to defined skills, abilities, and norms	Published research, position papers, practice papers, and evidence-based guidelines to practice
Education	Demonstrate competency at selected levels by meeting set criteria and passing credentialing exams	CADE Standards of Education; CDR Registration Examination for Dietitians
Autonomy	The profession is self-governing and independent in advancing practice	CDR Professional Development Portfolio Process
Service	Provide food and nutrition services for individuals and population groups and other stakeholders	Nutrition Care Process and Model; Nutrition Care Manual; Evidence-Based Guides to Practice

Adapted from Maillet JO, Skates J, Pritchett E. Scope of dietetics practice framework. *Journal of the American Dietetic Association* 2005;105(4):634–640.

communication, and biological, physiological, behavioral, and social sciences to achieve and maintain optimal human health" within flexible scope of practice boundaries to capture the breadth of the profession.[40] In the 1990s, dietetics began to define the unique competency of dietitians by using the term "medical nutrition therapy" (MNT) and promoting dietitians as its providers. MNT is defined as "nutritional diagnostic therapy and counseling services for the purpose of disease management which are furnished by a registered dietitian or nutrition professional."[41] Further, it is "a specific application of the nutrition care process in clinical settings that is focused on the management of diseases."[41]

MNT is provided by dietitians who work in a variety of clinical settings, including acute care, long-term care, private practice, and community and public health. Clearly describing MNT as its unique competency has distinguished dietitians from purveyors of food supplements and restaurateurs. It has also resulted in MNT being incorporated into several key pieces of legislation.[42,43]

Levels of Dietetic Practice: A Three-Tier System

To meet the needs of patients and clients in these diverse settings, dietetics is currently stratifying itself into three levels of professional practice. Specifically, Scope of Practice and Standards of Professional Performance documents describe generalist, specialist, and advanced practice.[27] To establish the credibility of these distinctions, each of these levels should be based on a defined structure that includes educational programs incorporating practice experience, a defined skill set, and credentials. The basis of these components is role delineation, task analysis, practice audit, or other formal research that supports a unique area of practice and set of skills that have multiple uses.

Figure 2–2 illustrates the roles of these components in developing practice. Figure 2–2 may also be applied to each of the three levels of practice discussed next.

Entry-Level Practice

Entry-level dietetics practice has been described using role delineation studies and practice audits.[9–12] Based on the most recent of these studies, the profession has confirmed that the first three years of practice constitute an entry-level period.[12] Entry-level competence in dietetics practice is based on standards of education that mandate a minimum of a baccalaureate degree accompanied by a minimum of

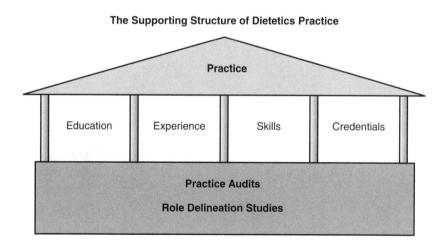

FIGURE 2–2 A Conceptual Representation of the Supporting Structure of Dietetics Practice

900 hours of supervised practice.[44] Because entry-level education and supervised practice must include broad competencies, dietitians may pass the registration exam for dietitians and enter the workforce with as little as one undergraduate-level course in MNT and as little as six to eight weeks of supervised MNT practice. On passing the Registration Exam for Dietitians, entry-level dietitians are considered competent to practice in the areas of entry-level food and nutrition, clinical and community nutrition, education, research, and food and nutrition systems and management.[45]

Based on the findings from several research studies, entry-level practice is defined as the first three years of practice. Dietitians may practice at this level as generalists for an entire career, or they may elect to move along a developing career continuum. Chambers et al. have identified changes that occur on the novice-to-expert continuum, as shown in Table 2–3.

Table 2–3 Conceptualization of Performance along the Novice-to-Expert Continuum

Novice	Beginner	Competent	Proficient	Expert
Rule driven				Schema driven
Rigid				Smooth, flexible
Slow				Efficient
Errors				Flawless
On request				Responsive to context
Extrinsic rewards				Intrinsic rewards
Performance separate from evaluation				Continuous self-monitoring
Teacher responsibility				Performer responsibility
Isolated performance segments				Integrated procedures
One task at a time				Multitasking
Surface features				Deep structure
One method				Choice
Dependent		Independent		Interdependent
Semiconscious		Conscious		Semiconscious
Poor content recall		Great deal of content recall		Reduced content recall

Adapted from Chambers DW, Gilmore CJ, Maillet JO, Mitchell BE. Another look at competency-based education in dietetics. *Journal of the American Dietetic Association* 1996;96(6):614–617.

Specialty Practice

Given the expanding knowledge in some areas of practice, dietitians with an interest in MNT may elect to deepen their knowledge in a single area of practice by narrowing their focus to specialty practice. The American Dietetic Association (ADA) defines specialty practice as "concentrating or delimiting one's focus to part of the whole field of dietetics (e.g., ambulatory care, long-term care, diabetes, renal, pediatric, private practice, community, nutrition support, research, sports nutrition)."[40] The ADA further states that "within the knowledge and skill hierarchy, specialty practice dietitians have acquired the proficient specialized knowledgebase, complex decision-making skills, and clinical competencies for specialty level practice, the characteristics of which are shaped by the context in which an RD [registered dietitian] practices."[27] At present, specialty credentials in medical nutrition therapy are available from the American Diabetes Association, the National Board of Nutrition Support Certification, and the Commission on Dietetic Registration.[46–48] A list of specialty credentials in MNT and the organizations sponsoring them appears in Table 2–4.

In its definition of specialty practice, the ADA is careful to state that specialty credentials are not necessary for specialty practice. This statement recognizes that there are specialties within dietetics with insufficient numbers of clinicians or the extensive knowledgebase required to support a specialty credential. Specialty credentials are typically awarded following documented practice experience and a credentialing exam. Specifications for these exams are based on role delineation studies and practice audits.[9–11] For some specialties, Standards of Practice and Standards of Professional Performance have been defined.[27,49,50] Notably, dietitians with specialty credentials often have unique job descriptions and job roles.[51]

Dietitians obtain the knowledge required to pass the credentialing exam by their own initiative, usually without benefit of accredited educational programs such as courses, residencies, or fellowships. Study guides are available for most specialty credentials, as are occasional review courses. Documented practice experience is a prerequisite for some, but not all, credentials.

Advanced Practice

As early as 1972, the ADA recommended that dietitians who had advanced professional education and/or professional training in responsible positions be eligible for certification through examination and review of advanced education and professional experience.[35] The first role delineation study, which was also conducted in 1972, was based on job descriptions compiled by the investigators.[52] Following its publication, a discussion of the need for advanced practice in management and

Table 2–4 Specialty Credentials in Medical Nutrition Therapy

Specialty Credential	Education Requirement	Experience Requirement	Test	Website
Board Certified Specialist in Pediatric Nutrition (CSP)	Baccalaureate degree and registered dietitian status for a minimum of three years	4000 hours of pediatric nutrition practice within the last five years	Yes	www.cdrnet.org
Board Certified Specialist in Renal Nutrition (CSR)	Baccalaureate degree and registered dietitian status for a minimum of three years	4000 hours of renal nutrition practice within the last five years	Yes	www.cdrnet.org
Board Certified Specialist in Sports Dietetics (CSD)	Baccalaureate degree and registered dietitian status for a minimum of three years	1500 hours of sports nutrition practice within the last five years[a]	Yes	www.cdrnet.org
Board Certified Specialist in Gerontological Dietetics (CGN)	Baccalaureate degree and registered dietitian status for a minimum of three years	4000 hours of renal nutrition practice within the last five years	Yes	www.cdrnet.org
Certified Nutrition Support Dietitian (CNSD)	RD credentialed as a registered dietitian	None[b]	Yes	www.nutritioncertify.org
Certified Diabetes Educator (CDE)	RD or master's degree in nutrition	1000 hours of diabetes education practice within the last five years	Yes	www.ncbde.org

a. Until May 31, 2009, education will be allowed to substitute for a maximum of 1200 hours of the required experience.

b. Two years experience is suggested.

clinical dietetics ensued, but the idea was rejected by the ADA's House of Delegates in 1979.[53,54]

More sophisticated methodology was applied in 1989, when Kane and colleagues conducted a task inventory analysis of practitioners that formed the basis of the first study of advanced practice.[9] In a follow-up study, Bradley et al. investigated how advanced practice dietitians performed (rather than which tasks were involved).[5] The Commission on Dietetic Registration used these studies to develop an advanced practice credential, the Fellow of the American Dietetic Association (FADA), though it was later discontinued for unknown reasons.[55]

Currently, the ADA defines advanced practice by stating that "the advanced practice dietitian is an RD who has acquired the expert knowledge base, complex decision-making skills, and clinical competencies for expanded practice, the characteristics of which are shaped by the context in which the RD practices"[27] The use of the word "expert" within this definition, compared with "proficient" in the definition of specialty practice, helps in clarifying the point that advanced practice dietitians have a higher level of skill than specialized dietitians. The ADA also recognizes a breadth of skill in stating that "advanced-level practice is characterized by the integration of a broad range of unique theoretical, research-based, and practical knowledge that occurs as a part of training and experience beyond entry level."[27]

At present, the single advanced practice credential available to dietitians practicing MNT is Board Certification in Advanced Diabetes Management (BC-ADM).[56] The profession of dietetics does not accredit advanced level dietetic education programs, although at least one such program is available.[57] To date, the profession has developed comprehensive Standards of Practice and Standards of Professional Performance documents that include advanced level performance indicators.[27,40,49,50] Interest in advanced practice persists, with the most recent advanced practice audit being completed in 2007.

The Difference Between Specialty and Advanced Practice

Close examination of the standards for the BC-ADM and Certified Diabetes Educator (CDE) reveals that a higher level of practice is required to qualify for the BC-ADM. Unique functions of the BC-ADM include physical assessment, regimen assessment and adjustment, therapeutic problem solving, and case management.[58] Table 2–5 provides specific examples of points at which the language describing advanced practice and specialty practice in terms of the task of care planning differs.

Table 2-5 Examples of Language Illustrating the Difference in Specialty and Advanced Practice

	CDE (Certified Diabetes Educator)[59]	BC-ADM (Board Certified Advanced Diabetes Manager)[58]
Care plan	Perform an individualized biopsychosocial and cognitive assessment of the individual with diabetes and/or the caregivers	Identify expected clinical outcomes derived from the assessment data and diagnosis/problem list, and individualize expected outcomes with the client, and with the health-care team when appropriate
	Dietitian Specialist in Behavioral Health[49]	**Advanced Practice Dietitian in Behavioral Health**
Nutrition diagnosis	Use specialty level clinical judgment skills (e.g., select from a range of possibilities with additional consideration of the client learning style; readiness and willingness to change)	Use advanced diagnostic reasoning and judgment (i.e., reflecting the holistic focus of behavioral health as a complex disorder)

For the CDE (a specialist), care planning is mentioned within the context of the caregiver and the individual with diabetes. No mention is made of collaboration with other professionals or caregivers to implement the plan. In contrast, the BC-ADM (an advanced level of practice) demonstrates a higher level of skill by predicting outcomes and interacting with the healthcare team as appropriate.

SUMMARY

Increasingly complex knowledge and skills are needed to practice advanced medical nutrition therapy (MNT). Although several studies document the existence of practice beyond the entry level, as yet no clear model of advanced medical nutrition therapy practice dietetics has been identified. Despite the fact that the nature of advanced practice skills and the methods by which they are acquired are not widely understood, dietitians practicing MNT need a clearly defined pathway from entry level to advanced practice to ensure that they will achieve credibility in the workplace. Studies of advanced practice have been complicated by two obstacles: The number of advanced practitioners is small, and these individuals are difficult to identify. The available studies suggest that certain skills constitute advanced practice, and with these findings it may be possible to predict an advanced practice model. Nevertheless, clear language is needed to describe the different level of practice. The profession has attempted to stratify itself into at least three distinct levels: entry level, specialty practice, and advanced practice. Given the stringent education and credentialing requirements in the health professions and the growing emphasis on scope of practice issues, it is unlikely that dietitians who lack formal advanced practice credentials will be widely accepted in health care.

KEY POINTS

- Advanced practice exists in many professions but it is difficult to describe.
- Descriptions of advanced practice in dietetics have focused on who advanced practice dietitians are rather than what they do.
- Specialty practice exists in many healthcare fields, but research suggests that specialty and advanced practice do not overlap.
- To increase advanced level dietitians' value in the marketplace, obtain reimbursement, and demonstrate outcomes, clearer descriptions of advanced practice are needed.

SUGGESTED READING

Benner PA. *From novice to expert: Excellence and power in clinical nursing practice.* Menlo Park, CA: Addison-Wesley, 1984.
Dreyfus HL, Dreyfus SE. *Mind over machine.* New York: Free Press, 1986.
Gladwell M. *Blink.* New York: Little, Brown, 2005.
Schon DA. *The reflective practitioner.* New York: Basic Books, 1983.

EXPERIENCES TO TRY

1. Describe what a mentor or colleague does that makes him or her an advanced practitioner. Write down this description, file it away, and, after finishing this book or course, reread it to see if your opinion has changed.
2. Describe what your job would look like if you were to implement an advanced practice MNT model in your current work setting or with your ideal job.

REFERENCES

1. Merriam-Webster Online. Available at www.m-w.com/. Accessed July 5, 2006.
2. Ericsson KA, Charness N, Feltovich PJ, Hoffman RR. *The Cambridge handbook of expertise and expert performance.* Cambridge, UK: Cambridge University Press, 2006.
3. Galton F. Hereditary genius. Macmillan and Company. Available at http://galton.org/. Accessed December 29, 2006.
4. Ericsson KA, Krampe RT, Clemmens T-R. The role of deliberate practice in the acquisition of expert performance. *Psychological Review* 1993;100(3):363–406.
5. Bradley RT, Young WY, Ebbs P, Martin J. Characteristics of advanced-level dietetics practice: A model and empirical results. *Journal of the American Dietetic Association* 1993; 93(2):196–202.
6. Dreyfus HL, Dreyfus SE. *Mind over machine.* New York: Free Press, 1986.
7. Gladwell M. *Blink.* New York: Little, Brown, 2005.
8. Lafferty LJ. Development of a methodology to determine and validate competency statements for dietitians employed in foodservice management positions at different levels of practice. Unpublished Dissertation, University of Missouri 1981.
9. Kane MT, Estes CA, Colton DA, Eltoft CS. Role delineation for dietetic practitioners: Empirical results. *Journal of the American Dietetic Association* 1990;90(8):1124–1133.
10. Kane MT, Cohen AS, Smith ER, Lewis C, Reidy C. 1995 Commission on Dietetic Registration: Dietetics practice audit. *Journal of the American Dietetic Association* 1996; 96(12):1292–1301.
11. Rogers D, Leonberg BL, Broadhurst CB. 2000 Commission on Dietetic Registration: Dietetics practice audit. *Journal of the American Dietetic Association* 2002;102(2): 270–292.
12. Rogers D, Fish JA. Entry-level dietetics practice today: Results from the 2005 Commission on Dietetic Registration entry-level dietetics practice audit. *Journal of the American Dietetic Association* 2006;106(6):957–964.e922.
13. Sprately E, Johnson A, Sochalski J, Fritz M, Spencer W. The registered nurse population: Findings from the national sample survey of registered nurses. Available at www.bhpr.hrsa.gov/healthworkforce/reports/rnsurvey/rnss1.htm. Accessed January 7, 2007.
14. MacKle TJ, Touger-Decker R, Maillet JOS, Holland BK. Registered dietitians' use of physical assessment parameters in professional practice. *Journal of the American Dietetic Association* 2003;103(12):1632–1638.
15. Cresci G. Dietitians place feeding tubes? *Nutrition* 2002;18(9):778–779.
16. Brody RA, Touger-Decker R, Von Hagen S, Maillet JOS. Role of registered dietitians in dysphagia screening. *Journal of the American Dietetic Association* 2000;100(9): 1029–1037.
17. Mueller CM, Colaizzo-Anas T, Shronts EP, Gaines JA. Order writing for parenteral nutrition by registered dietitians. *Journal of the American Dietetic Association* 1996;96(8): 764–768.
18. Olree K, Skipper A. The role of nutrition support dietitians as viewed by chief clinical and nutrition support dietitians: Implications for training. *Journal of the American Dietetic Association* 1997;97(12):1255–1260.
19. Silver H, Wellman N. Nutrition diagnosing and order writing: Value for practitioners, quality for clients. *Journal of the American Dietetic Association* 2003;103(11):1470–1472.

20. Moreland K, Gotfried M, Vaughn L. Development and implementation of the clinical privileges for dietitian nutrition order writing program at a long-term acute-care hospital. *Journal of the American Dietetic Association* 2002;102(1):72–74.

21. Wildish DE. An evidence-based approach for dietitian prescription of multiple vitamins and minerals. *Journal of the American Dietetic Association* 2004;104(5):779–786.

22. Drug Enforcement Administration. Mid-level practitioners authorization by state. Available at http://www.deadiversion.usdoj.gov/drugreg/practioners/index.html. Accessed January 9, 2007.

23. Bowen JL. Educational strategies to promote clinical diagnostic reasoning. *New England Journal of Medicine* 2006;355(21):2217–2225.

24. Skipper A, Lewis NM. A look at the educational preparation of the health diagnosing and treating professions: Do dietitians measure up? *Journal of the American Dietetic Association* 2005;105(3):420–427.

25. Beck CT. Trends in nursing education since 1976. *MCN American Journal of Maternal and Child Nursing* 2000;25(6):290–295.

26. American Nurses Association. Social policy statement for nursing. Available at www.ana.org. Accessed November 29, 2003.

27. Kulkarni K, Boucher JL, Daly A, et al. American Dietetic Association: Standards of practice and standards of professional performance for registered dietitians (generalist, specialty, and advanced) in diabetes care. *Journal of the American Dietetic Association* 2005;105(5):819–824, 824e.811–824e.822.

28. Hamric AB, Spross JA, Hanson CM (eds.). *Advanced nursing practice*, 2nd ed. Philadelphia: W. B. Saunders, 2000.

29. Bradley RT. Fellow of the American Dietetic Association credentialing program: Development and implementation of a portfolio-based assessment. *Journal of the American Dietetic Association* 1996;96(5):513–517.

30. Center for Medicare and Medicaid Services. Conditions of participation for hospitals. Available at http://www.cms.hhs.gov/CFCsAndCoPs/06_Hospitals.asp#TopOfPage. Accessed November 28, 2006.

31. Druss BG, Marcus SC, Olfson M, Tanielian T, Pincus HA. Trends in care by nonphysician clinicians in the United States. *New England Journal of Medicine* 2003;348(2):130–137.

32. Hodges PA. Perspectives on history: Military dietetics in Europe during World War I. *Journal of the American Dietetic Association* 1993(8);93:897–900.

33. Isch C. A history of hospital fare. *Journal of the American Dietetic Association* 1964;45:441–446.

34. Erickson-Weefrs S. Past, present, and future perspectives of dietetics practice. *Journal of the American Dietetic Association* 1999;99(3):291–293.

35. American Dietetic Association. *The profession of dietetics: The report of the 1972 Study Commission on Dietetics*. Chicago: American Dietetic Association, 1972.

36. Bistrian BR, Blackburn GL, Hallowell E, Heddle R. Protein status of general surgical patients. *Journal of the American Medical Association* 1974;230(6):858–860.

37. Bistrian BR, Blackburn GL, Vitale J, Cochran D, Naylor J. Prevalence of malnutrition in general medical patients. *Journal of the American Medical Association* 1976;235(15):1567–1570.

38. Institute of Medicine. *Health professions education: A bridge to quality*. Washington, DC: Institute of Medicine, 2003.

39. U.S. Department of Labor, Bureau of Labor Statistics. Health diagnosing and treating practitioners. Available at http://www.bls.gov/oco/ocos077.htm. Accessed January 6, 2007.

40. Kieselhorst K, Skates J, Pritchett E. American Dietetic Association: Standards of practice in nutrition care and updated standards of professional performance. *Journal of the American Dietetic Association* 2005;105(4):614–645, 645.e611–245.e610.

41. Lacey K, Pritchett E. Nutrition care process and model: ADA adopts road map to quality care and outcomes management. *Journal of the American Dietetic Association* 2003;103(8):1061–1071.

42. Smith RE, Patrick S, Michael P, Hager M. Medical nutrition therapy: The core of ADA's advocacy efforts (Part 1). *Journal of the American Dietetic Association* 2005; 105(5):825–834.

43. Smith RE, Patrick P, Michael P, Hager M. Medical nutrition therapy: The core of ADA's advocacy efforts (Part 2). *Journal of the American Dietetic Association* 2005;105(6): 987–996.

44. Bruening KS, Mitchell BE, Pfeiffer MM. 2002 accreditation standards for dietetics education. *Journal of the American Dietetic Association* 2002;102(4):566–577.

45. Registration examination for dietitians. *Commission on Dietetic Registration.* Available at http://www.cdrnet.org/certifications/rddtr/rdcontent.htm. Accessed January 4, 2007.

46. National Certification Board for Diabetes Educators. 2006 certification handbook for diabetes educators. Available at http://www.ncbde.org/certhandbook_app.html. Accessed April 21, 2006.

47. Professional Testing Corporation. Examination for Nutrition Support Dietitians; Handbook for candidates. Available at http://www.nutritioncertify.org/exams/DIET 2006.pdf. Accessed November 9, 2006.

48. CDR certifications. Available at http://www.cdrnet.org/certifications/index.htm. Accessed January 1, 2007.

49. Emerson M, Kerr P, Soler MDC, et al. American Dietetic Association: Standards of practice and standards of professional performance for registered dietitians (generalist, specialty and advanced) in behavioral health. *Journal of the American Dietetic Association* 2006;106(4):608–613, 613.e601–613.e623.

50. Robien K, Levin R, Pritchett E, Otto M. American Dietetic Association: Standards of practice and standards of professional performance for registered dietitians (generalist, specialty, and advanced) in oncology nutrition care. *Journal of the American Dietetic Association* 2006;106(6):946–951.e921.

51. American Dietetic Association. *Job descriptions: Models for the dietetics profession.* Chicago: American Dietetic Association, 2003.

52. Baird SC, Wenberg, BG. Investigator shares methodology for first role delineation studies. *Journal of the American Dietetic Association* 1995;95(11):1257.

53. American Dietetic Association. *Report of the House of Delegates ad hoc committee to study the feasibility of establishing board certification for specialist groups.* Chicago: American Dietetic Association, 1976.

54. American Dietetic Association. *Report of the House of Delegates ad hoc committee to set up framework for which specialty boards could be established and to suggest minimum standards and guidelines for specialty boards and for selecting members.* Chicago: American Dietetic Association, 1977.

55. Bogle ML, Balogun L, Cassell J, Catakis A, Holler H, Flynn C. Achieving excellence in dietetics practice: Certification of specialists and advanced-level practitioners. *Journal of the American Dietetic Association* 1993;93(2):149–150.
56. Valentine V, Kulkarni K, Hinnen D. Evolving roles: From diabetes educators to advanced diabetes managers. *Diabetes Educator* 2003;29(4):598–610.
57. Touger-Decker R. Advanced-level practice degree options: Practice doctorates in dietetics. *Journal of the American Dietetic Association* 2004;104(9):1456–1458.
58. Board Certified–Advanced Diabetes Management. Available at http://www.diabetes educator.org. Accessed February 1, 2007.
59. Martin C, Daly A, McWhorter L, Schwide-Slavin C, Kushion W. The scope of practice, standards of practice, and standards of professional performance for diabetes educators. *Diabetes Educator* 2005;31(14):487–512.

A Model for Advanced Medical Nutrition Therapy Practice

"When we mean to build, we first survey the plot, then draw the model; and then we see the figure of the house . . ."—William Shakespeare

The dietetics profession has defined advanced practice, and named some advanced practice skills in the recent Scope of Practice Documents.[1] However, a clear picture of what the advanced practice dietitian knows or does is not widely understood or agreed upon by practicing dietitians. Having a clear vision of advanced medical nutrition therapy (MNT) practice is an important beginning for dietitians who wish to increase their skills. Descriptions of advanced practice may then be aggregated into useful benchmarks for dietitians who wish to expand their practice.

In the past, the author of this book has identified advanced practice dietitians who are working in MNT and interviewed a number of them for a research project designed to identify what advanced practice dietitians do. This research has revealed common knowledge and activities of advanced practitioners, which are depicted in the model discussed in this chapter.[2] The chapter also contains many direct quotes used by dietitians to describe their practice. At the end of the chapter is an exhibit from an advanced practice dietitian. The purpose of this chapter is to help make the vision of advanced practice more concrete by providing a model and descriptions based on actual practice.

AN ADVANCED PRACTICE MODEL

To better understand what advanced practice dietitians do, Skipper and Lewis studied the skills of these healthcare professionals.[2] They selected a sample of credentialed advanced practice dietitians with expertise in MNT from a variety of practice settings, clinical specialties, and geographic locations. These dietitians participated in in-depth interviews concerning their job responsibilities, career paths, and practice activities. Transcripts of the interviews provided a rich database of information describing advanced MNT practice.

An analysis of the hundreds of pages of data from the interview transcripts resulted in the Using Initiative to Achieve Autonomy model, which is shown in Figure 3–1. This model is based on an overarching theme plus five sub-themes that apply to patients, practice, and the practice environment. The overarching theme incorporates two characteristics of advanced practitioners: initiative and autonomy. The five sub-themes that emerged from the data were labeled aptitude, attitude, context, expertise, and approach.

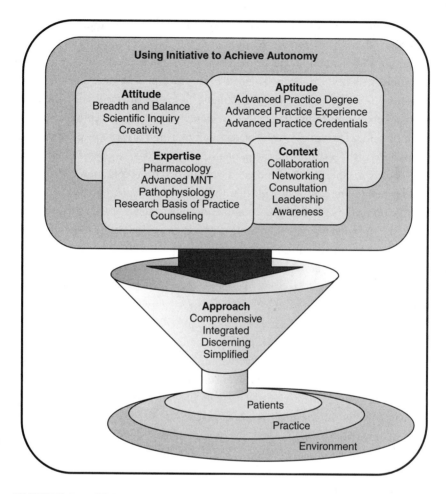

FIGURE 3–1 Using Initiative to Achieve Autonomy: A Model of Advanced Medical Nutrition Therapy Practice

Source: Skipper A, Lewis NM. Using initiative to achieve. *Journal of the American Dietetic Association* 2006; 106:1219–1225. Copyright Elsevier (2006).

Initiative and Autonomy

A definition of initiative that seems to describe the advanced practice interviewees is "at one's own discretion; independently of outside influence or control."[3] Study participants exhibited initiative in several ways.

For example, these dietitians took responsibility for their own practice. Personal ownership of their practice was obvious even though the dietitians worked in tightly regulated environments that were heavily controlled with policies, procedures, protocols, and standards. These dietitians acknowledged regulation, but were not constrained by it. They recognized their ability to initiate and influence care by developing and changing regulations. These dietitians used initiative to develop and implement new protocols designed to improve patient care. They changed practice as needed to meet changing demands. One dietitian initiated interventions for her clients, stating that "It was wrong to practice in a receptive way, waiting to be told what to do." Another dietitian used initiative to improve patient care, stating that "Not hurting the patient isn't enough—my job is to help make things better for the patient," and cited examples of protocols and programs designed to streamline care or provide new therapies. A third dietitian described herself as action oriented and "not complaining, but wanting to fix things." As a result, she initiated a broader role for dietitians in a dialysis center to include nutrition-related medication management.

Interviewees maintained both career and work agendas, and saw themselves as directing their own agendas. One dietitian sought increasingly challenging positions in her successful quest to earn a six-figure salary within 10 years of graduation, stating that it was necessary "not to accept self-imposed restrictions, but to believe in herself, not to make the minimum her ceiling." Another saw herself and other advanced practice dietitians as shaping and defining their own career ladders rather than merely climbing a career ladder determined by someone else. Dietitians with initiative functioned especially well in solo practice settings or as members of a multidisciplinary group of practitioners.

Autonomy, which is defined as "the quality or state of being self-governing," was often a result of initiative.[3] Several changes in health care have pointed to the need for more autonomous practitioners. As healthcare delivery moves outside the traditional hospital environment, autonomous practice is becoming the norm for an increasing number of practitioners from all health professions. More care is being delivered in private practice, outpatient clinics, and the community, where fewer physicians or managers are available to directly supervise dietitians. A growing number of dietitians are also functioning independently or in environments where the details of care are decided collaboratively.

While remaining grounded in dietetics, most interviewees had moved beyond traditional roles and structures. In fact, movement from a traditional role, job, or department was often cited as a prerequisite or parallel to advanced MNT practice. One dietitian moved into the nursing department to facilitate initiatives that were "too scary" for the dietary department in her hospital. Another dietitian established a new department within her hospital to distinguish the MNT focus of dietitians from the catering and foodservice satisfaction focus of the foodservice department.

Several worked in nontraditional settings or had assumed nontraditional activities. Others moved into private practice or joint practice with a physician group so as to establish an autonomous practice. Some functioned as solo practitioners with total responsibility for nutrition therapy but also were responsible for nutrition policy within a multidisciplinary setting. One dietitian successfully convinced a nationally known physician to hire her rather than a nurse as manager of his newly established clinic. In that role, she developed patient care protocols, trained patients in diabetes self-management, and hired and trained nurses, encouraging them to become credentialed in diabetes education.

Several dietitians exercised a commitment to autonomy even when that commitment required sacrifice. One dietitian was so strongly committed to autonomy that she declined referrals from a physician who limited the services she provided to his patients. Another obtained advanced practice nursing credentials to facilitate autonomous practice because she "did not want to be a puppet." A third dietitian reflected on her decision to obtain a physician assistant credential, stating that "I wanted to be able to continue to manage patients independently. So it was really more autonomy and to know more about medicine."

The most frequently cited hallmark of autonomous practice was the ability to independently order, modify, and monitor MNT. Several dietitians had obtained clinical privileges to order parenteral and enteral nutrition, diets, and laboratory tests, or to modify medications such as insulin, phosphate binders, and iron supplements. Clinical privileges to modify drug doses or order nutrition interventions were viewed as an important mechanism that allowed dietitians to use their advanced skills and knowledge to provide improved care. Clinical privileges were also viewed as a mechanism to achieve parity in the practice setting. In the words of one interviewee, "Order writing goes a long way toward raising the public image of any profession . . . I think if they see you as someone who has some sort of autonomy over some issues . . . it gives you a lot more legitimacy with everyone—the general public [and] the medical profession."

A benefit of the increased responsibility associated with clinical privileges was increased professional and job satisfaction. Interviewees accepted the additional responsibility associated with autonomous practice because it was a more satisfying means to provide better care to their patients. The autonomy component was supported by behaviors including a sense of practice ownership. That is, these dietitians recognized that they owned their practice and accepted responsibility to practice from a broader perspective than a single patient interaction. They used initiative to identify where they could make a difference, and then implemented practices, programs, and behaviors that supported those differences.

Aptitude

The sub-themes begin with aptitude, which encompasses the educational and experiential background of the advanced practice dietitian. This preparation is sometimes documented with a formal credential or, much more often, with a portfolio of advanced practice experience and accomplishments. Thus the aptitude sub-theme was composed of the education, credentials, and experience needed for advanced practice.

Interviewees uniformly expressed the need for graduate-level education as a prerequisite to practice. At the same time, they expressed a strong need for more clinically focused education. Dietitians were aware of the growing trend toward increased education in other health professions and clearly stated that current educational programs in dietetics need to be strengthened to prepare advanced practice dietitians. Dietitians also noted that an advanced degree was one of the elements distinguishing advanced practice from specialty practice.

Dietitians recognized the need for substantial experience as a prerequisite for advanced practice. While most agreed that at least five to seven years of practice experience was needed, at least one stated that she was "still fresh" after 10 years in renal and diabetes practice in a major academic medical center. Other credentials mentioned as prerequisites to advanced practice included certification, publications, presentations, volunteer leadership opportunities, and program development. The need for credentials to document specific, marketable skills—rather than recognition of achievement or service—was viewed as essential. There was uniform agreement that education alone, even at the practice doctorate or Ph.D. level, was insufficient and that persons with an advanced degree could not be considered advanced level practitioners unless they had several years of practice experience.

Attitude

The attitude sub-theme incorporates frequently mentioned skills that fuel initiative. It is characterized by a breadth and balance of perspective, scientific inquiry, and creativity. Breadth and balance of perspective is used as a criterion to distinguish between specialty and advanced practice: The specialist has depth of knowledge in a narrow area, whereas the advanced practitioner brings a breadth of knowledge to the practice setting. Examples of inquiry were expressed on two levels. Advanced practice dietitians often consulted the scientific literature to find solutions to clinical problems. They also asked probing questions about clinical and nutritional problems with respect to individual patients and groups of patients. A third characteristic of advanced practice dietitians was the creativity that they relied on to innovate and survive.

Context

The context sub-theme refers to the skills needed for autonomous practice and to the relationship between advanced practitioners and their environment. The interviewed dietitians participated in interdisciplinary collaboration, expressing the need to be connected with others caring for their patients, sharing in joint decision making, and contributing their expertise to a group of healthcare professionals. Advanced practice dietitians also maintained large networks of colleagues both within their own profession and within other professions. Some advanced practice dietitians functioned in a consultative role, sharing their expertise with others as requested. They used leadership to shape their environment to change practice. They did all this with a sense of timing and knowledge of how their activities fit within the larger context, a characteristic named awareness.

Expertise

Expertise contains the skills needed as the basis of advanced practice. When applied by the advanced practice dietitian, it is the expertise subsection that results in increased value in the marketplace. As expected, many advanced practice dietitians demonstrated expertise in a particular area of dietetics. They easily discussed the most complex and difficult of cases, spontaneously giving rich examples of sophisticated interventions. More than once, they mentioned uncovering facts or solving problems after others had tried and failed. Specific topics of expertise that recurred throughout the interviews included nutritional pharmacology, advanced MNT, pathophysiology, the research or evidence supporting practice, counseling theory and skills, and medical co-morbidities prevented or treated with nutrition intervention.

Approach

Each of the first four sub-themes is populated with the knowledge, skills, practitioner characteristics, and expertise that the advanced practice dietitian brings to practice. Components of the aptitude, attitude, context, and expertise sub-themes serve as background for the advanced practice dietitian in the approach to practice depicted in the funnel portion of Figure 3–1. Advanced practice dietitians exhibited a comprehensive, integrated, discerning, yet simplified approach to information that could be instantly shifted to meet the needs of the situation at hand. The model also incorporates the ease with which advanced level practitioners constantly processed, reformatted, and added to the depth and breadth of their knowledge and skill. Finally, the ripples at the bottom of the model represent individual patients, groups of patients that may be called a practice, and the larger environment the advanced practice dietitian affects.

The advanced practice dietitians interviewed for the study exhibited all of the characteristics depicted in the model, suggesting that the model should be viewed as a whole rather than as a series of separate pieces. There is no indication that any one sub-theme is more important than another. It is likely that advanced dietetics practice will resemble the Using Initiative to Achieve Autonomy model, but validation studies are needed for confirmation. In addition, advanced practice dietitians might possess other skills or characteristics that were not identified in this preliminary study, so ongoing research in this area is encouraged.

The findings of Skipper and Lewis complement—rather than contradict—existing data concerning advanced practice. If these findings are applied to Bradley's model and incorporated into the ADA's definition of advanced practice, the result might look something like the framework depicted in Table 3–1. Combining these two sources provides a more robust model and begins to provide some information for practitioners interested in developing their skills, or for educators wishing to offer educational programs.

Based on the findings of Skipper and Lewis, an addition to the ADA definition of advanced practice is also proposed. The recent definition developed by the ADA's quality management committee was "expert knowledgebase, complex decision-making skills, and clinical competencies for expanded practice, the characteristics of which are shaped by the context in which an RD practices." This definition further refers to expanded and specialized knowledge, skills, competencies, and experience. Based on the results of their research, Skipper and Lewis proposed that the definition be changed to reflect the fact that the RD shapes the practice context rather than practicing according to the context.[2]

Advanced and Specialty Practice

Earlier role studies differentiated between specialty and advanced practice,[4,5] and nothing in the work of Skipper and Lewis would appear to alter this conclusion. However, in the workplace, confusion sometimes arises regarding the difference in advanced and specialty practice. The ADA has differentiated specialty and advanced practice according to Dreyfus and Dreyfus's stages of expertise, assigning the word "proficient" to the specialty practitioner and reserving the word "expert" for

Table 3–1 A Revised Definition and Core Competencies for Advanced Practice Dietitians

Proposed Changes to Advanced Practice Dietetics

Definition

An RD who has acquired the expert knowledgebase, complex decision-making skills, and clinical competencies for expanded practice, *and who has the skills to shape the context in which the RD practices*[2]

Practitioner Characteristics[2,4]

Advanced Practice Degree

Advanced practice experience

Advanced practice credentials

Approach to practice

   Comprehensive

   Integrated

   Discerning

   Simplified

Core Competencies[2]

   Expertise

   Nutrition pharmacology

   Advanced medical nutrition therapy

   Nutrition pathophysiology

   Research basis of practice

   Counseling

   Co-morbidities

Attitudinal competencies

   Breadth and balance of perspective

   Scientific inquiry methods

   Creativity

Contextual competencies

   Collaboration

   Networking

   Consultation

   Leadership

   Awareness

Note: Words in regular type were found in the work of Bradley et al. Words in italics are from the work of Skipper and Lewis.

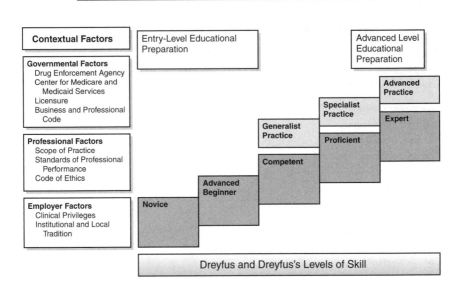

FIGURE 3–2 The Pathway to Advanced Medical Nutrition Therapy Practice

the advanced practice dietitian. It appears that three levels of dietetics practice exist: entry-level, specialty, and advanced practice (Figure 3–2).

APPLICATION TO PRACTICE

Dietitians may have difficulty relating to the model in Figure 3–1 for two reasons. First, the model is an abstract representation of concepts described with nonclinical wording. Exhibit 3–1 is included here to help translate the model into a more realistic clinical situation. Reading the exhibit and answering the accompany questions should assist in visualizing what an advanced practice dietitian does.

Second, the model does not provide specific facts or formulas that a dietitian must know to be considered an advanced level practitioner. Instead, the themes function as categories of knowledge or skills. More detail about the themes and sub-themes will be included in subsequent chapters of this book.

EXHIBIT 3–1

An Advanced Practice Dietician at Work

From outside the door of the ICU, I recognized a distinctive odor and deduced that we had a GI bleeder on the unit. The gastroenterologist was conferring with the ICU attending outside room 236, which confirmed the location. The name on the board was unfamiliar, meaning the patient had been admitted overnight.

As I approached the unit clerk's desk, I noticed a request to type and cross match two units of blood for the patient. Pointing to the paperwork, I asked how long the patient had been on the unit. "Came over from rehab about 1:00 A.M.," was the reply. "He already got two units and GI's been in there most of the night." "Any family here?" I asked. The unit clerk rolled her eyes in the direction of the lounge, where I had seen several well-dressed men and women hovering around an elderly woman. I would need to talk to them, as I was unlikely to get any information from the patient. "Has surgery been here?" I asked. "The residents were here about an hour ago." "Have they asked for a surgical ICU reservation?" I asked. The unit clerk shook her head, "Not yet."

In the medical ICU, things change quickly. You have to adapt. For a GI bleeder, the treatment approach is a major factor in how we manage nutrition. If GI can control the bleeding with cautery, the patient will eat. If the bleeding worsens and the patient must undergo surgery, I would place a nasointestinal tube postoperatively. With massive bowel resection or severe malnutrition, the patient might need parenteral nutrition. In any case, we would begin a work-up and adapt our plan to the patient's condition.

Our nutrition fellow appeared from the back of the unit, where she had been rounding with the ICU team. We'd started the fellowship several years before for pharmacists, dietitians, and physicians. It was fun working with them.

The fellow began: "The new patient is a 79-year-old male patient of Dr. Rothman who came over last night from ortho rehab. He is 5 feet 9 inches.

continues

EXHIBIT 3–1 *continued*

His ideal weight is 160 pounds, but he weighs 183 pounds now. So he needs about 25 calories per kilogram and 1.2 grams of protein per kilogram to give about 2000 to 2100 calories and 100 grams of protein per day per unit protocol. His prior medical history includes an appendectomy and cholecystectomy years ago. He was admitted 8 days ago with a fractured hip. His cholesterol is high, and so is his BUN. Everything else is normal. The ICU residents want to start a tube feeding. We should recommend a renal formula at 40 mL/hr via a PEG tube."

"Oh, does he have a PEG?" I asked.

"No, but I think they should place one," the fellow replied, "so we can use his GI tract."

"Well, let's take a minute to see what's going on," I said. "Could you check his baseline renal function?" I knew that a PEG was probably not an option at this time, and made a note to review enteral access with the fellow later today.

Moving toward the room, I glimpsed the patient through a crack in the curtains. He was pale and the shape of his belly suggested more generalized edema than ascites. Still, it would be nice to know if he had liver disease or if the bleeding was from something else. Drips and blood were hanging. The GI attending was in the room, which this late in the year suggested that the problem was serious enough that the fellow had called for backup.

I sidled into the room, took a quick look at the medications, IVs, and monitors. The patient was on D5.45 at 175 mL per hour. The monitor showed mean arterial pressure that was a little lower than we liked for enteral feeding, and the patient's PCO_2 was marginal, but his cardiac output was adequate. Enteral feeding was a judgment call. If he stopped bleeding, the mean arterial pressure would rise, but then he would also be able to eat. Two lumens of a triple-lumen catheter were being used; the third port was capped. As long as anesthesia didn't contaminate the third port in the operating room, parenteral nutrition would be an easy option if the patient went to surgery. Intake and output was 3 liters positive since midnight, but the pa-

EXHIBIT 3–1 *continued*

tient's urine output was adequate, which meant that we wouldn't be limited in the volume of feeding we could give.

I returned to the nursing station and quickly checked the midnight labs. PT and PTT were normal, so liver disease probably wasn't the source of the bleeding. Electrolytes were normal, but as expected the BUN was high, with the creatinine just at the high end of normal. Given the patient's age and the antibiotic regimen associated with hip reduction surgery, this was no surprise. The fellow was searching for baseline labs so that we could assess the change in his renal function over time. However, with a BUN out of proportion to creatinine and adequate urine output, it was likely that the BUN was elevated due to bleeding. I made a note to ask whether the fellow understood the issue and how to assess it.

The only remaining question was the treatment plan. The patient probably hadn't eaten much in the 8 days since his admission. He would have been NPO for surgery and likely missed meals because of physical therapy and pain. We were running out of time before his lack of nutrient intake would begin to negatively affect his prognosis. Since it was Thursday, it would be better to get something started today rather than tomorrow. That way, we'd be at goal before the weekend.

At that point, the surgery resident walked into the unit. His body language told me that the patient was going to the OR. I looked down the hall and saw the attending talking to the family, which confirmed my thinking. The intern stopped at the desk and asked the clerk to make a surgical ICU reservation. "What's he going for?" I asked. "AVM resection" was the reply. "Okay, so he's been without food for most of the last 8 days. Should we start something, or wait and see how things go in the OR?" I knew better than to suggest feeding tube placement during the case. To do so would merely prolong the OR time and increase the risk of postoperative complications. The choices were to start PN or place a tube in the next day or so.

continues

EXHIBIT 3–1 *continued*

At that point, the attending appeared and asked me if we could start PN tonight. "Of course," I replied, "unless you want to wait until tomorrow and I'll place a tube."

"Well, we could, but in a patient this age, I'm not sure about the blood supply to his gut."

"Right," I said, thinking of the mean arterial pressure. "Why don't we start PN so that he can get some nutrition, then transition to EN or oral as he stabilizes? He really needs to be fed, so I'll get a liter up to the surgical ICU for you tonight."

"Thanks," the attending replied.

I asked the fellow to calculate a liter of PN formula with half of goal dextrose in it.

"What about refeeding?" she asked.

"We're going to put enough phosphorus in his PN so that it doesn't drop," I replied.

"Shouldn't we limit the dextrose to 2.5/mg/kg/min?" she asked.

"We could take that approach, but since we are managing his electrolytes, it won't be necessary," was my reply. "Instead, we'll advance him according to a protocol we developed based on a randomized trial we did here a few years ago. There's a copy of our paper in your readings. You might want to take a quick look at it so you'll know what we're doing tomorrow."

ICU = intensive care unit; GI = gastrointestinal; BUN = blood urea nitrogen; PEG = percutaneous endoscopic gastrostomy; IV = intravenous; PCO$_2$ = partial carbon dioxide concentration; OR = operating room; PN = parenteral nutrition; PT = prothrombin time; PTT = partial thromboplastin time; NPO = nil per os (nothing by mouth); AVM = aortovenous malformation; EN = enteral nutrition.

SUMMARY

Advanced practice skills have been difficult to define and describe. Bradley et al. identified some practitioner characteristics such as a master's degree that were associated with advanced practice.[4,6] The Using Initiative to Achieve Autonomy model contains five sub-themes that add to the understanding of the skills that advanced practice dietitians use. The skills of the advanced practice dietitian are broad, whereas the skills of the specialist appear narrower, suggesting differences in the two levels of practice.

KEY POINTS

- Interviews with advanced practice dietitians yielded valuable information that has been analyzed and used to describe the skills of advanced practice dietitians. The resulting model, called Using Initiative to Achieve Autonomy, contains five sub-themes: attitude, aptitude, expertise, context, and approach. These sub-themes are, in turn, applied to patients, practice, and the practice environment.
- The model provides a richer picture of advanced medical nutrition therapy practice than was previously available. The model can be validated using further qualitative research or using quantitative methods.

SUGGESTED READING

Schwide-Slavin C. Case study: A patient with type 1 diabetes who transitions to insulin pump therapy by working with an advanced practice dietitian. *Diabetes Spectrum* 2003;16:37–40.

EXPERIENCES TO TRY

Read the exemplar and/or the suggested reading. Then answer the following questions.

1. Can you find an example where the speaker illustrates her knowledge of the context of care and uses it to adapt the intervention?

2. Can you find an example where the speaker uses trends rather than analyzing single events or pieces of information to make decisions?

3. Can you find an example where the speaker uses data to confirm rather than form impressions?

4. Read through the exemplar again and identify sentences or phrases that fit with the various parts of the model. Can you can identify examples of any of the following:

   Collaboration

   Consultation

   Co-morbidities

   Pathophysiology

   Research basis of practice

5. Take a look at Figure 3–2. Where do you think the speaker in the exhibit is on the continuum?

REFERENCES

1. Maillet J, Skates J, Pritchett E. American Dietetic Association: Scope of dietetics practice framework. *Journal of the American Dietetic Association* 2005;105(4):634–640.
2. Skipper A, Lewis NM. Using Initiative to Achieve Autonomy: A model for advanced medical nutrition therapy practice. *Journal of the American Dietetic Association* 2006; 106(8):1219–1225.
3. Merriam-Webster Online. Available at www.m-w.com/. Accessed July 5, 2006.
4. Bradley RT, Young WY, Ebbs P, Martin J. Characteristics of advanced-level dietetics practice: A model and empirical results. *Journal of the American Dietetic Association* 1993;93(2):196–202.
5. Kane MT, Estes CA, Colton DA, Eltoft CS. Role delineation for dietetic practitioners: Empirical results. *Journal of the American Dietetic Association* 1990;90(8):1124–1133.
6. Bradley RT, Ebbs P, Martin J. Specialty practice in dietetics: Empirical models and results. *Journal of the American Dietetic Association* 1993;93(2):203–210.

Aptitude

"One can never consent to creep when one feels an impulse to soar." —*Helen Keller*

Aptitude has been defined as a "natural or acquired disposition or capacity for a particular purpose, as, oil has an aptitude to burn."[1] The dietitian may have a natural capacity for advanced practice. However, as noted in Chapter 2, in a complex healthcare profession, the acquisition of skills through education and practice is needed to develop the confidence required to establish credibility. Indeed, the three components of aptitude—education, practice experience, and credentials—are so widely used in health care as to be considered almost essential.

In dietetics, mechanisms to obtain advanced practice education, experience, and credentials are not well established. As advanced medical nutrition therapy (MNT) practice emerges, however, the details of advanced education, practice experience, and credentials will inevitably be developed. Likewise, the structure and content of advanced practice education will be defined. The nature and duration of supervised practice will be agreed upon, and residency or fellowship programs implemented. Credentialing mechanisms will be developed.

This chapter discusses the aptitude portion of the advanced MNT model. In addition, an educational and credentialing system is proposed. The chapter also presents suggestions for individuals to obtain advanced practice skills in areas where definitions of education, experience, and credentialing programs are not yet available.

BRIEF REVIEW OF ENTRY-LEVEL PREPARATION

The current system of dietetic education was developed in 1927.[2] At that time, the basic qualifications for dietetic education were a minimum of a baccalaureate degree, followed by six months (900 hours) of supervised practice experience. In the 1960s, the dietetics profession implemented the Dietetic Registration examination for dietitians and the registered dietitian (RD) credential as a means to ensure competency to practice dietetics.[3] Thus entry-level dietetics practice is based on education, practice, and a credential.

Entry-Level Education

The baccalaureate dietetics degree typically incorporates about two years of general education courses, such as those in mathematics, science, humanities, accounting, computer science, and business. It also requires completion of courses designed to provide the foundation knowledge and skills needed to support practice. A typical list of undergraduate dietetics courses appears in Table 4–1. This table illustrates the breadth of dietetics education requirements needed to meet the accreditation standards promulgated by the Commission on Accreditation of Dietetics Education.[4]

The supervised practice portion of dietetics education is designed to allow students to apply knowledge gained in the classroom to the actual work setting. During supervised practice (also called a dietetic internship or clinical portion of a coordinated program), students are guided by experienced mentors or preceptors through rotations that vary according to program goals, resources, and available facilities. Thus supervised practice tends to focus on one of the traditional divisions of dietetics, such as clinical or community nutrition. An example of the distribution of internship across a breadth of required topics is found in Table 4–2.

Tables 4–1 and 4–2 provide insight into the duration and depth of classroom learning and practice experience in MNT. While some accredited dietetics education programs may offer or even require additional coursework, it is clear that

Table 4–1 Typical Undergraduate Dietetics Curriculum

Course	Number of Credits
Basic Foods	4
Cultural Foods	4
Foodservice Management	4
Foodservice	4
Basic Nutrition	4
Community Nutrition	4
Nutrition Evaluation	4
Medical Nutrition Therapy	4
Advanced Nutrition	4
Total	36

Table 4–2 Example of Supervised Practice Rotations

Rotation	Hours
Orientation	40
Clinical (e.g., acute and long-term care)	320
Foodservice	280
Community (e.g., ambulatory clinic and public health)	200
Staff Relief	80
Total	920

Table 4–3 Content Specifications for the Registration Exam for Dietitians

Content Area	Percentage of Questions
Food and Nutrition Science	12%
Nutrition Care Process and Model: Complex Conditions	40%
Counseling, Communication, Education, and Research	10%
Foodservice Systems	17%
Management	21%

Source: Commission on Dietetic Registration. Available at www.cdrnet.org. Accessed October 4, 2007.

dietitians may enter the workforce with as few as three or four college credits in MNT and as few as 8 to 10 weeks of practice delivering MNT.

Entry-Level Credentials

Upon their satisfactory completion of an accredited dietetics education program, graduates must pass the registration exam to become registered dietitians.[5] The content outline for the Dietetic Registration exam (Table 4–3) reflects the breadth of the dietetics profession. The RD credential certifies competence to practice dietetics at the entry level, which is defined as the first three years of practice.[6] To maintain the RD credential, dietitians must obtain continuing education related to specific goals they establish.

Tables 4–1, 4–2, and 4–3 reveal the breadth of topics incorporated into undergraduate education and entry-level credentialing for dietitians. After completing this broad education, the overwhelming majority of dietitians enter the workforce in clinical or community settings, where they work directly with patients or clients to improve their health by implementing MNT.[6] Given the increasing complexity of MNT, some critics have pointed out the need for additional MNT education.[7] The availability of additional, advanced education in MNT is justified based on our increasing knowledge of the effects of nutrition on the disease process and new findings related to the influence of diet on many disease processes, and the need to develop new nutrition interventions and test their effectiveness.

REVIEW OF ADVANCED PRACTICE EDUCATION

To provide a framework for the discussion of educational preparation for advanced practice, it is useful to briefly review the types of academic degrees available to dietitians. The baccalaureate degree required of dietitians is the first of a series of academic degrees. It is aligned in stepwise fashion with the master of science (M.S.) and doctor of philosophy (Ph.D.) degrees. According to the U.S. Department of Education, the baccalaureate degree is awarded for four years of post-secondary or college-level study.[8] The master's degree is awarded for successful completion of one or two years of full-time, college-level study beyond the baccalaureate degree and denotes mastery of a particular subject area. The Ph.D., which is the highest academic degree, requires mastery of a field of knowledge and demonstrated ability to extend that knowledge by performing scholarly research. Obtaining a Ph.D. typically takes at least three years of full-time study. The B.S.–M.S.–Ph.D. degree sequence is designed to support an academic career in teaching or, following completion of a postdoctoral fellowship, research. Such an academic career path is chosen by fewer than 5% of dietitians, however.

For complex or higher-risk professions, such as law, medicine, or pharmacy, additional education and training are needed to demonstrate entry-level competency. In these professions, students obtain a baccalaureate degree first, and then are admitted to a first professional degree program (e.g., law school, medical school, or pharmacy school).[8] The first professional degree is bestowed upon completion of the academic requirements for beginning practice in a given profession and demonstration of a level of professional skill beyond that normally required for a bachelor's degree.

In some professions (e.g., social work and occupational therapy), the first professional degree is granted at the master's level. In others (e.g., pharmacy, medicine, and law), the first professional degree is a doctoral-level degree. The first professional degree may also be called a practice doctorate, clinical practice doctorate, clinical doctorate, or professional doctorate degree. It is usually awarded following completion of a program that requires four academic years of college-level education prior to admission, is three to four years long, and blends didactic or classroom and supervised practice instruction to produce an entry-level practitioner with both a sufficient academic background and practice-based skills.[8]

Educational Systems in Other Health Professions

As health professions have become more complex, the educational requirements to enter professional practice have steadily increased:

- The physical therapy profession developed the doctor of physical therapy (DPT) degree and ceased accreditation of baccalaureate degrees in physical therapy in 2002.[9] Students pursuing a physical therapy degree may choose between a master's degree and a DPT degree.

- The pharmacy profession originally conceived the doctor of pharmacy (Pharm.D.) degree as an advanced practice degree for registered pharmacists, but it became a first professional degree.[10] Pharmacy ceased accreditation of baccalaureate programs and moved exclusively to the first professional degree in 2004.[11]
- The American Occupational Therapy Association ceased accreditation of baccalaureate programs in January 2007.[12,13] Occupational therapists may be credentialed at the entry level after obtaining a master or doctor of occupational therapy degree.
- Speech-language pathologists have traditionally used the M.S. degree as the entry-level credential. However, the audiology portion of this profession has initiated the doctor of audiology (Aud.D.). By 2012, applicants for the Certificate of Clinical Competence in Audiology must have a doctoral degree.[14]

These examples demonstrate a clear trend toward graduate degrees as preparation for entry-level practice. This trend has extended to dietitians, where a major report on dietetics education has advocated entry-level dietetics preparation at the master's level.[7] Besides dietetics, the only other health diagnosing and treating profession that does not use graduate entry-level preparation is nursing.

While most health professions have moved toward reducing the types of educational programs, the nursing profession has taken a different approach. It uses three different routes to entry-level practice: a three-year diploma program, a two-year associate degree, or a four-year baccalaureate degree.[15] The master of science in nursing (M.S.N.) has been used as the educational requirement for advanced nursing practice.[16] This professional degree is used to prepare advanced practice nurses (i.e., clinical nurse specialists, nurse practitioners, certified registered nurse anesthetists, and the majority of nurse midwives). Completion of the M.S.N. is typically followed by 500 hours of supervised practice and a credentialing exam in a specialty practice area.

The nursing profession has recommended changing to the doctor of nursing practice (DNP) degree for preparation of advanced level nursing practitioners.[17] This degree is designed to prepare clinical practice scholars who practice a skill set beyond what basic level nurses are licensed to perform. This change has not yet been accepted, but is recommended for implementation by 2012.[18]

Dietetics Education Compared to Education for Other Professions

In the majority of health diagnosing and treating professions, advanced education is a prerequisite for entry-level practice.[19] Figure 4–1 provides a comparison of the entry-level educational requirements for several of these professions. It clearly shows a gap in the level of educational preparation between dietitians and other health professionals. From Figure 4–1, it is clear that professions with greater authority, responsibility, reimbursement, and economic status require a master's or doctoral degree and at least a year of supervised practice before entry into the profession. In addition, it is clear that dietitians receive less education and practice experience than all of the health diagnosing and treating professions except nurses.

Currently, dietitians practicing MNT typically seek an M.S. degree in nutrition because the subject matter is more closely related to MNT than other available degrees. However, traditional M.S. degree programs are designed to produce graduates who have mastered basic science and research skills as a step in the progression to a Ph.D. and a career in teaching and research. We do not know whether these degrees contain the practice-based coursework and experience needed to enhance MNT skills. A few dietitians obtain other degrees, such as the master of education (M.Ed.) or master of counseling. Unfortunately, these degrees do not typically provide the advanced MNT knowledge necessary to meet the needs of an increasingly sophisticated patient population and healthcare system.

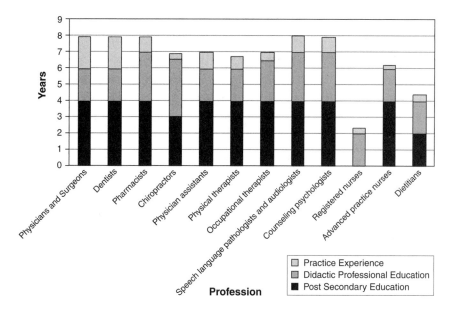

FIGURE 4–1 Duration of Typical Post-Secondary, Didactic Professional Education, and Supervised Practice Required for Entry into Selected Health Diagnosing and Treating Professions[2,20–29]

A few graduate-level programs in MNT or clinical nutrition have been established to work in conjunction with the supervised practice experience required to enter professional practice as a registered dietitian. A comparison of curricula for a traditional Master's and a clinical Master's degree is found in Table 4–4. It is unknown how often or even if it is possible for practicing clinicians to access these programs. Given that these degrees are associated with entry-level preparation, we do not know whether they include advanced practice experiences and courses. While an advanced practice master's degree in MNT could be developed, it would be difficult to use as a tool for differentiation in a marketplace where more than 40% of dietitians already have a master's degree.

Recently, a task force appointed by the ADA's House of Delegates recommended that a master's degree become the standard for entry-level dietetics.[7] If this recommendation is accepted by the profession, the distinction between an entry-level and advanced practice master's would become even more difficult to define. Thus it is reasonable to explore the feasibility of a practice doctorate degree in dietetics, clinical nutrition, or MNT.

A Description of a Medical Nutrition Therapy Practice Degree

A practice-based doctorate degree in MNT or clinical nutrition could meet the needs of dietitians interested in obtaining advanced practice skills. Although the practice doctorate degree for dietitians was first proposed in 1993, it is unknown whether such programs were developed at that time.[30] Results of recent research studies suggest that both baccalaureate- and master's-prepared dietitians with four or more years of experience are interested in enhancing their MNT knowledge and skills even further and, therefore, are interested in clinical doctorate degrees.[31]

Table 4–4 Comparison of a Traditional and Clinical Master of Science Degree in Nutrition

Course Topics	Traditional Master of Science	Clinical Master of Science
	Number of Credits	
Nutrition specialization	18	15
Supervised clinical practice-residency	0	6
Research	6	3
Research project	3	3
Elective	3	3
Total credits	30	30

Based on the Using Initiative to Achieve Autonomy model discussed in Chapter 3, a list of skills and courses for such a degree was developed (see Table 4–5). The items on this list were incorporated into a survey of more than 1000 clinical dietitians and clinical nutrition managers. Dietitians who responded to the survey were most interested in courses that would improve their skill in direct patient or client care. Likewise, employers in academic medical centers were interested in hiring dietitians with skills derived from the courses shown in Table 4–5. By contrast, graduate program directors were less interested in offering these courses. Nevertheless, several institutions have discussed offering a practice doctorate degree.

Existing Educational Programs

At least one doctor of clinical nutrition degree program has been developed and began enrolling students in 2003.[32,33] This program is designed for experienced, M.S.-prepared, registered dietitians. It is offered almost entirely online. Because this program is housed within an interdisciplinary college of health professions,

Table 4–5 Courses Preferred by Clinical Dietitians and Their Managers in Academic Medical Centers

Course	Credits
Advanced medical nutrition therapy	4
Nutrition disease state management	4
Nutrition tests and procedures	2
Evidence-based nutrition diagnosis	2
Nutrition pathophysiology	8
Advanced counseling skills	3
Nutrition pharmacology	4
Advanced supervised practice	6
Completion of a clinical nutrition outcome research project	6
Clinical nutrition outcome research methods	6
Professional nutrition communication	3
Practice management	2
Advanced practice roles	2
Advanced practice role transformation	2
Total	54

Source: Skipper A, Lewis NM. Clinical dietitians, employers, and educators are interested in advanced practice education and professional doctorate degrees in clinical nutrition. *Journal of the American Dietetic Association* 2006;106(12):2062–2066.

students may take advantage of interdisciplinary courses in nutrition-related topics, such as pharmacology and pathophysiology. Table 4–6 highlights the differences between the professional doctorate degree and the Ph.D. degree curriculum.

In the future, traditional Ph.D. programs could be adapted to meet the need for advanced practice education. Opportunities exist for traditional Ph.D. programs to incorporate practice-based experiences and research, assuming resources and faculty interest allow for this expansion. Ultimately, combined faculties might be used to develop programs, and technology could be used to support them. In an era when health care is being delivered or supported by technology, distance learning might readily be employed to assemble visiting faculty members or clinical experts to lead discussions, provide input into projects, or discuss cases. Indeed, dietitians who learn via distance learning may find it easier to adapt to technology in the workplace.

Education: A Summary

Clearly, progress is being made toward the education of advanced practice dietitians. Nevertheless, it remains unknown whether traditional institutions of higher learning will adapt so as to meet the educational needs of dietitians or whether alternatives such as online educational programs provided by proprietary universities will provide advanced practice education in MNT. How successful the educational programs are in the long run will depend on how successful their graduates are in securing advanced practice positions. Until such programs become widely available, dietitians may choose to educate themselves by undertaking structured read-

---

Table 4–6 Comparison of the Course Requirements for the Doctor of Philosophy versus the Practice Doctorate

Course Credits	Doctor of Philosophy	Practice Doctorate
	Number of Credits	
Nutrition specialization	15–18	33
Supervised clinical practice-residency	0	5 (450 hours)
Research	12	6
Research project	15 dissertation credits	6–9 outcomes research credits
Other	15–18	0
Total credits	60	51

Source: Touger-Decker R. Advanced practice doctorate in clinical nutrition. *Topics in Clinical Nutrition* 2005;20(1):48–53.

ing and continuing education programs. They may also wish to investigate a variety of online courses as means to improve their expertise.

REVIEW OF ADVANCED PRACTICE EXPERIENCE

Experience may be defined as "having firsthand knowledge of a particular situation."[34] Health professions rely heavily on supervised practice experience to teach diagnoses and interventions for specific patient populations. These supervised practice experiences provide the opportunity for dietitians to observe expert practitioners and to model their behaviors. Practice also contributes to confidence. Not surprisingly, dietitians consider learning by practicing to be the most valuable educational form.[35]

Learning by Experience

The advanced practice learning experience for dietitians should provide opportunities for dietitians to practice advanced MNT interventions with patients. This experience should also provide opportunities for students to observe role models for advanced practice behaviors. While advanced practice students may wish to focus their experience on a specific patient population or type of intervention, the experience should also provide ample opportunities to develop and practice collaboration, consultation, scientific inquiry, leadership, awareness, and other skills in addition to developing MNT expertise.

Advanced practice experience is usually gained during residency programs. Such a residency typically involves supervised practice of about one year's duration.[36,37] Although fellowships are also used for practice experience, they are typically two years in duration and incorporate a year of clinical or laboratory research.[36,37] Dietetics has defined the term "residency" as meaning a planned educational program following published guidelines for specialty training that includes didactic and supervised experiential learning.[38] In particular, guidelines for such programs in metabolic nutrition care and pediatrics have been developed.[38,39]

Some reports have indicated the development of advanced practice residencies and fellowships in some areas of dietetics.[39,40] While these programs may be accredited by other agencies, the Commission on Accreditation of Dietetics Education has not developed an accreditation mechanism for dietetic residencies or fellowships. The need for accredited residency or fellowship training in dietetics has been studied, but advanced practice residencies have not been developed on a large scale.[41]

Acquiring Expertise

Advanced level practitioners are considered expert performers of their profession.[42] The acquisition of expertise—which is key to achieving this advanced level of practice—has been the object of intense study and discourse.[43] The methods used by experts to acquire their skills have been studied in professions as diverse as mathematics, sports, medicine and surgery, accounting, and theater. It is generally agreed that it takes a long and intense period of study to acquire expertise. It is also generally agreed that experts consciously participate in the advancement of their skills through both formal education and intense practice. Whether or not formal supervised practice programs are available, dietitians will need to be proactive in establishing advanced practice expertise. The following discussion is intended to stimulate thinking about how dietitians might develop advanced practice skills.

A key factor in developing expertise is reflection. Epstein and Hundert recognized this critical need for reflection when they defined professional competence as "the habitual and judicious use of communication, knowledge, technical skills, clinical reasoning, emotions, values, and reflection in daily practice for the benefit of the individual and community being served."[44] Dietitians will have been exposed to reflection as part of the process required to maintain the RD credential. In this process, dietitians are asked to think about the skills they currently have as well as the skills they wish to develop in the future.

Shöen provides an expanded exploration of reflection in his classic text on the topic.[45] He uses the term "reflective practice" to describe the differences in the ways in which novices and experts complete their work.[45] Expert practitioners can reflect while in action, changing and adapting their approaches within an evolving situation. According to Shöen, to develop this skill practitioners should identify positive experiences and reflect on how to create similar situations, identify areas of ignorance and learn to ask for help in those areas, and find and push the limits of risk.

Another tool in acquiring expertise is deliberative practice.[46] In an extensive review of the literature and their own experiments, Ericsson and colleagues found that experts spent more time in practicing their skills than their non-expert colleagues and worked to meet specific goals each week. In some fields, experts used activities designed to improve performance of tasks that could be mastered sequentially.[46] In dietetics, the models of advanced practice could be used to guide reflection on needed skills. Dietitians might then work with mentors to design practice

Table 4–7 Ericsson et al.'s Theoretical Framework for Deliberative Practice

Resources

Deliberative practice requires available time for and energy for the individual as well as access to teachers, training materials, and training facilities.

Motivation

Deliberative practice is motivated by further achievements in performance.

Effort

Deliberative practice is effortful and is sustained for a limited amount of time before exhaustion.

Source: Ericsson KA, Krampe RT, Clemmens T-R. The role of deliberate practice in the acquisition of expert performance. *Psychological Review* 1993;100(3):363–406.

experiences that improve skills based on Ericsson et al.'s findings. Ericsson et al.'s framework for the acquisition of expert performance provides some insight into how expertise may be achieved. Table 4–7 shows this theoretical framework for deliberative practice as a method for acquisition of expertise.

Experience: A Summary

Practice-based experience is a powerful and popular learning tool. Notably, mentored practice is widely used in health care as means to perfect skills. The lessons of such experiential learning can be enhanced with deliberate practice and reflection to set goals and develop a plan to identify and improve needed skills. Until structured residency or fellowship programs become more widely available, individual dietitians are encouraged to use reflection and deliberative practice to develop their expertise. Of course, not all experience will contribute to learning: It is essential that reflection be used to identify needed skills, and practice applied to perfect those skills. Clearly, more opportunities are needed for dietitians to interact with mentors and to learn new skills.

ADVANCED DIETETICS PRACTICE CREDENTIALS

The National Organization for Competency Assurance defines "credential" as "the umbrella term that includes the concepts of accreditation, licensure, registration, and professional education."[47] In health care and dietetics, credentials are used to demonstrate competence to practice in a particular profession. Credentials are designed to protect the public from unqualified practitioners who may not have the knowledge or skill to perform in a safe manner. The purpose of credentials is to establish criteria for fairness, quality, competence, and/or safety for professional services provided by authorized individuals for products or for educational endeavors. Typically, awarding of credentials is based on a standardized demonstration of knowledge via a written or oral exam, observation of skills performed, or a portfolio of work.

Following the role delineation studies of the late 1980s, the dietetics profession developed an advanced practice credential, the Fellow of the American Dietetic Association (FADA).[48] To earn this credential, advanced practice dietitians were required to write a response to a professional scenario. In addition, applicants supplied information about job and other professional responsibilities that demonstrated advanced practice. Candidates submitted portfolios that were graded by a review panel according to stringent criteria. More than 350 dietitians were awarded the FADA. After a few years, however, this credential was changed from a competency credential to a recognition credential and was closed to new members.

Currently, only one advanced practice credential is available to the registered dietitian: the Board Certified–Advanced Diabetes Management (BC-ADM) credential. This multidisciplinary credential is also available to nurses and pharmacists.[49] To be eligible for the BC-ADM, a dietitian must obtain a master's degree related to dietetics and document 500 hours of experience in diabetes practice prior to taking an examination. Details of the activities required to obtain the BC-ADM are found in Table 4–8.

Table 4–8 Competency and Scope of Practice for Board Certified–Advanced Diabetes Management

---

The Advanced Practitioner in Diabetes Management has an advanced degree and is able to

· Perform complete and/or focused assessment,
· Recognize and prioritize complex data in order to identify needs of patients with diabetes across the life span; and
· Provide therapeutic problem solving, counseling, and regimen adjustment.

The scope of advanced clinical practice includes management skills such as medication adjustment, medical nutrition therapy, exercise planning, counseling for behavior management, and psychosocial issues. Attaining optimal metabolic control may include treatment and monitoring of acute and chronic complications. The depth of knowledge and competence in advanced clinical practice and diabetes skills affords an increased complexity of decision making, which expands the traditional discipline-specific practice. Research, publications, mentoring, and continuing professional development are expected skill sets.

Source: American Association of Diabetes Educators. Available at http://www.diabeteseducator.org. Accessed September 19, 2007.

Interest in advanced dietetics practice has continued to grow, and the Commission on Dietetic Registration conducted an audit to describe advanced practice in dietetics in 2007. This activity provides evidence that there is an effort under way to measure advanced practice in dietetics. Depending on the results of the audit, the dietetics profession may again develop an advanced practice credential. In the interim, dietitians will need to develop and document their own credentials. They can do so by using samples of work in a professional portfolio. Such a portfolio may include a variety of information—for example, exemplars of situations, descriptions of practice activities, papers, projects, and numbers and types of cases managed and their outcomes.

SUMMARY

Three types of evidence—background education, experience, and credentials—are needed to establish credibility as an advanced practice dietitian. The desired program for preparing advanced practice dietitians in MNT is a practice doctorate degree. As part of this degree, an advanced practice dietitian should obtain sufficient practice experience to become confident in the advanced practice role. In addition, a credential is needed that demonstrates competence in skills of value to employers. For advanced practice to be implemented consistently, widespread agreement is needed on this pathway.

KEY POINTS

- Many dietitians with a master's degree obtained this degree as part of their entry-level education experience. A master's degree is unlikely to be sufficient to distinguish the advanced practice dietitian in the healthcare marketplace, however, given that more than 40% of all dietitians have a master's degree.
- Experience is a critical component of advanced practice. It provides dietitians with opportunities to develop and hone a breadth and depth of advanced practice skills.
- Credentials demonstrating advanced practice may be offered by organizations or, if they are unavailable, may be documented by practitioners themselves in the form of a portfolio.

SUGGESTED READING

Ericsson KA, Charness N, Feltovich PJ, Hoffman RR. *The Cambridge handbook of expertise and expert performance.* Cambridge, UK: Cambridge University Press, 2006.

Schon DA. *The reflective practitioner.* New York: Basic Books, 1983.

EXPERIENCES TO TRY

1. Review Figure 4–1 and list the professions. Conduct informal conversations with members of these professions in which you discuss the level or reimbursement, autonomy to make clinical decisions, and authority to prescribe drugs or other medical treatment that they have or that their colleagues have. Find out which procedures they perform and then try to correlate their activities with the level of education shown in the diagram.

2. Develop a means of reflecting on your practice. Spend a few minutes each week in a quiet place and review the activities for the week that went well and those that did not. Can you make a plan for how to improve your performance? Can you identify resources or mentors that might help you improve your skills? Would regular journal reading or a journal club help to develop your practice skills?

3. Select an aspect of your practice that you would like to develop. Formulate a plan for developing that aspect of practice. Review the plan with a mentor and implement it using the methods suggested by Ericsson and Schon.

4. Review Exhibit 4–1 and reflect on whether you could develop a portfolio based on the advanced practice model described in Chapter 3.

EXHIBIT 4–1

Creating a Portfolio of Credentials

Beth was interested in developing an advanced practice position in her institution. She realized that she would have to demonstrate to her boss that she has different credentials than the entry-level and specialty dietitians in her institution. Beth's boss was supportive, but needed documentation of Beth's skills to reclassify her position.

EXHIBIT 4–1 *continued*

Beth was familiar with the professional development portfolio used to main-tain dietetic registration. She decided to apply the concepts in that portfo-lio to her own situation. She set aside a Sunday afternoon to think about her work. To jog her memory, Beth collected her most current curriculum vitae, recent performance evaluations, a file of letters she had collected from grateful patients and colleagues, and other documents that reminded her of positive job performance. She also obtained a copy of her employer's mission, vision, and values statement. Next, Beth reviewed the information in Table 3–1 and began to think both about her practice and about how her many activities could be organized according to current advanced practice models.

Beth realized that she had accomplished a great deal in the previous two or three years and would need to carefully design her portfolio to avoid over-whelming anyone who reviewed it. She decided to focus on the skills that were most consistent with her employer's objectives of improved patient care and reduced costs. Beth developed an outline for her portfolio, and then began to collect documents that she wanted to include in the portfolio.

Beth's curriculum vitae was several pages long, so she decided to edit it to resume form, eliminating all but the most recent advanced practice activi-ties. Beth had finished a master's degree program years before, but had re-cently entered into an advanced practice doctorate program. She listed the topics of the nutrition-related courses that she had completed, which in-cluded a course in the economics of medical nutrition therapy. She reviewed her recent productivity reports and briefly summarized her patient experi-ence terms of patient days, because her administrators used patient days as a measure of productivity. Her institution had adopted the Nutrition Care Process and Standardized Language, which made it easy for Beth to iden-tify the unique interventions she had performed and quantify the positive outcomes she had obtained.

Beth was certified in her specialty practice area and remembered to list that certification as well as a certificate she had earned in a non-dietetics-related

continues

EXHIBIT 4–1 *continued*

area that was important to her employer's organizational goals. With the one-page resume in draft form, Beth turned her attention to the next items for her portfolio.

First, Beth reflected on her practice philosophy. Only then did she begin to write down some ideas about her responsibility to her patients, her colleagues, and her employer. For example, she had always been a regular reader of two nutrition journals and one medical journal, so she incorporated reading into her practice philosophy, and made notes on two examples of how she applied research results to improve nutrition interventions in her patient population. She soon had a ¾-page draft describing her approach to her work and career. She laid the draft aside and noted on her calendar a time to come back and revise it.

Next, Beth began to think about ways to document that she had the necessary advanced practice attitude, context, and approach. She decided to use exemplars of her practice to document her skills. After studying the sub-themes in the advanced practice attitude, context, and approach categories, she decided to develop two exemplars: one that would relate to patient care and encompass the approach sub-theme, and another that would describe the results of a collaborative project that she had just completed with her colleagues in her assigned area of practice. She made notes for each exemplar, and resolved to work on developing these documents during the next week.

On the following Sunday afternoon, Beth developed one exemplar and revised the draft of her practice philosophy. That week she shared the practice philosophy with a pharmacist colleague and a senior colleague in the practice doctorate program. The third Sunday afternoon she wrote and revised the second exemplar and revised her practice philosophy based on feedback from her colleagues.

Beth assembled the resume, practice philosophy, exemplars, a summary of data from a recent outcomes measurement project, and an article she had written into a notebook for her boss to review. After making a few changes suggested by her boss, Beth and her boss wrote an advanced practice posi-

EXHIBIT 4–1 *continued*

tion description. They arranged meetings with the appropriate administrators to obtain approval of the position description and used the portfolio to compare Beth's activities to those of advanced practitioners from other professions to justify an appropriate salary.

REFERENCES

1. Brainy quote. Available at http://www.brainyquote.com/. Accessed March 13, 2007.
2. Commission on Accreditation of Dietetics Education. *Accreditation Handbook.* Chicago: American Dietetic Association, 2002.
3. CDR certifications. Available at http://www.cdrnet.org/certifications/index.htm. Accessed January 1, 2007.
4. Bruening KS, Mitchell BE, Pfeiffer MM. 2002 accreditation standards for dietetics education. *Journal of the American Dietetic Association* 2002;102(4):566–577.
5. Bogle ML. Registration: The sine qua non of a competent dietitian. *Journal of the American Dietetic Association* 1974;64(6):616.
6. Rogers D, Fish JA. Entry-level dietetics practice today: Results from the 2005 Commission on Dietetic Registration entry-level dietetics practice audit. *Journal of the American Dietetic Association* 2006;106(6):957–964.e922.
7. American Dietetic Association. Dietetics Education Taskforce report and recommendations. Available at http://www.eatright.org/ada/files/FINALDietEdTaskForceReport 22105.doc. Accessed June 7, 2006.
8. U.S. Department of Education, Institute of Educational Studies. Digest of educational statistics 2002. Available at http://nces.edu.gov/pubs. Accessed August 10, 2003.
9. American Physical Therapy Association. Doctor of physical therapy (DPT) degree frequently asked questions. Available at http://www.apta.org. Accessed June 29, 2006.
10. Marx MA. Pharmaceutical education: A matter of degree. *Annals of Pharmacotherapy* 1992;26:1000–1001.
11. American Council on Pharmaceutical Education. Implementation procedures for accreditation standards and guidelines for the professional program in pharmacy leading to the doctor of pharmacy degree. Available at www.acpe-accredit.org/docs/pubs. Accessed July 20, 2003.
12. Runyon CP, Aitken MJ, Stohs SJ. The need for a clinical doctorate in occupational therapy (OTD). *Journal of Allied Health* 1994;23(2):57–63.
13. American Occupational Therapy Association. Frequently asked questions regarding occupational therapy education. Available at http://www.aota.org/nonmembers/area2/links/links/link01.asp. Accessed June 22, 2006.
14. Nodar RH. New audiology certification standards: What they mean to you. *ASHA* 1999;4(3)1:8.
15. Beck CT. Trends in nursing education since 1976. *MCN American Journal of Maternal and Child Nursing* 2000;25(6):290–295.

16. Hamric AB, Spross JA, Hanson CM (eds.). *Advanced nursing practice*, 2nd ed. Philadelphia: W. B. Saunders, 2000.

17. AACN. Position statement on the practice doctorate in nursing. Available at http://www.aacn.nche.edu/DNP/DNPFAQ.htm. Accessed December 12, 2006.

18. American Association of Colleges of Nursing. *The essentials of doctoral education for advanced nursing practice*. Available at http://www.aacn.nche.edu/DNP/pdf/Essentials.pdf. Accessed July 24, 2007.

19. Skipper A, Lewis NM. A look at the educational preparation of the health diagnosing and treating professions: Do dietitians measure up? *Journal of the American Dietetic Association* 2005;105(3):420–427.

20. Liaison Committee on Medical Education. Function and structure of a medical school: Standards for accreditation of medical education programs leading to the MD degree. Available at http://www.lcme.org. Accessed June 11, 2006.

21. Commission on Dental Accreditation. Accreditation standards for advanced education programs in general dentistry. Available at http://www.ada.org. Accessed June 11, 2006.

22. Accreditation Council for Pharmacy Education. Accreditation standards and guidelines for the professional program in pharmacy leading to the doctor of pharmacy degree. Available at http://www.acpe-accredit.org/standards/default.asp. Accessed June 2, 2006.

23. Council on Chiropractic Education. Standards for doctor of chiropractic programs and requirements for institutional status. Available at http://www.cce-usa.org/. Accessed November 14, 2003.

24. Accreditation Review Commission on Education for the Physician Assistant. Accreditation standards for physician assistant education. Available at http://www.aapa.org. Accessed June 11, 2006.

25. American Physical Therapy Association. 2006 CAPTE Accreditation Handbook. Available at http://www.apta.org/AM/Template.cfm?Section=CAPTE1&TEMPLATE=cm/contentDisplay.cfm&CONTENTID=35141. Accessed January 23, 2007.

26. Accreditation Council for Occupational Therapy Education. Standards for an accredited educational program for the occupational therapist. Available at http://www.aoanet.org. Accessed November 14, 2003.

27. Council on Academic Accreditation in Audiology and Speech-Language Pathology. Standards for the certificate of clinical competence in audiology. Available at http://www.asha.org/about/credentialing/accreditation/accredmanual/. Accessed June 11, 2006.

28. American Psychological Association. Guidelines and principles for accreditation of programs in professional psychology. Available at http://www.apa.org. Accessed June 11, 2006.

29. Commission on Collegiate Nursing Education. Standards for accreditation of baccalaureate and graduate nursing programs. Available at http://www.aacn.nche.edu. Accessed November 15, 2003.

30. Christie BW, Kight MA. Educational empowerment of the clinical dietitian: A proposed practice doctorate curriculum. *Journal of the American Dietetic Association* 1993;93(2):173–176.

31. Skipper A, Lewis NM. Clinical dietitians, employers, and educators are interested in advanced practice education and professional doctorate degrees in clinical nutrition. *Journal of the American Dietetic Association* 2006;106(12):2062–2066.

32. Touger-Decker R. Advanced-level practice degree options: Practice doctorates in dietetics. *Journal of the American Dietetic Association* 2004;104(9):1456–1458.

33. Touger-Decker R. Advanced practice doctorate in clinical nutrition. *Topics in Clinical Nutrition* 2005;20(1):48–53.
34. Merriam-Webster Online. Available at www.m-w.com/. Accessed July 5, 2006.
35. Barr AB, Walters MA, Hagan DW. The value of experiential education in dietetics. *Journal of the American Dietetic Association* 2002;102(10):1458–1460.
36. Anonymous. Residencies? Fellowships? What's the difference??? Available at http://www.apta.org. Accessed November 28, 2003.
37. Anonymous. Definitions of pharmacy residencies and fellowships. *American Journal of Hospital Pharmacy* 1987;44(5):1142–1144.
38. American Dietetic Association. Guidelines for the development of residency programs in metabolic nutrition. Chicago: American Dietetic Association, 1995.
39. Coffey A, Compher C. Advanced dietetic training in nutrition support and metabolism: The University of Pennsylvania Medical Center experience. *Nutrition* 1996;12(11): 836–838.
40. McCoy BL, Balmer D. Development of a pediatric residency program for registered dietitians. *Journal of the American Dietetic Association* 1997;97(8):892–893.
41. Olree K, Skipper A. The role of nutrition support dietitians as viewed by chief clinical and nutrition support dietitians: Implications for training. *Journal of the American Dietetic Association* 1997;97(12):1255–1260.
42. Benner PA. *From novice to expert: Excellence and power in clinical nursing practice.* Menlo Park, CA: Addison-Wesley, 1984.
43. Ericsson KA, Charness N, Feltovich PJ, Hoffman RR. *The Cambridge handbook of expertise and expert performance.* Cambridge, UK: Cambridge University Press, 2006.
44. Epstein RM, Hundert EM. Defining and assessing professional competence. *Journal of the American Medical Association* 2002;287(2):226–235.
45. Schon DA. *The reflective practitioner.* New York: Basic Books, 1983.
46. Ericsson KA, Krampe RT, Clemmens T-R. The role of deliberate practice in the acquisition of expert performance. *Psychological Review* 1993;100(3):363–406.
47. Durley CC. *The NOCA guide to understanding credentialing concepts.* Washington, DC: National Organization for Competency Assurance, 2005.
48. Bradley RT. Fellow of the American Dietetic Association credentialing program: Development and implementation of a portfolio-based assessment. *Journal of the American Dietetic Association* 1996;96(5):513–517.
49. Certificate in childhood and adolescent weight management. Available at www.cdrnet .org/whatsnew/childhood.htm. Accessed March 26, 2004.

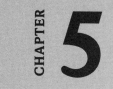

CHAPTER 5

Attitude

"Bite off more than you can chew, then chew it." —*Ella Williams[1]*

The attitude theme was the name given by advanced practice dietitians to a group of three sub-themes: scientific inquiry, creativity, and breadth and balance of perspective. One definition of attitude refers to a mental position, or feeling of emotion with regard to a fact or state.[2] Advanced practice dietitians frequently have a mental position that includes an organized or scientific and inquiring attitude. They are not bound by rules, but rather call on creativity to deal with situations. Advanced practice dietitians use their breadth and balance of perspective to develop medical nutrition therapy (MNT) that works for the patient.

This chapter provides a definition, description, and discussion of each of the attitude sub-themes. For dietitians wishing to increase their understanding of these sub-themes, exhibits are offered. Additional readings and skill-building exercises are also included to stimulate thinking and practice.

SCIENTIFIC INQUIRY

"There are two ways to slide easily through life: to believe everything or to doubt everything. Both ways save us from thinking." —*Alfred Korzybski[3]*

Scientific inquiry has been defined as an examination into facts or principles.[2] Interviews with advanced practice dietitians conducted by the author of this book revealed a common thread of curiosity expressed in a questioning yet scientific approach that is shared by these professionals. Advanced practice dietitians most often mentioned using scientific inquiry to solve patient-specific problems. In addition, they use an organized, scientific approach to develop solutions to common clinical and administrative problems, to research questions, and to develop new interventions or other services.

Advanced practice dietitians uniformly expressed the need for comprehensive and current knowledge not only in nutrition, but also in other advances related to their practice area. These professionals were knowledgeable, read widely, and were able to critique and selectively apply research literature located in nutrition and dietetics publications and medical journals. Not surprisingly, then, advanced practice dietitians have generated research questions and participated in clinical research studies that answer these questions. They have also used inquiry techniques to better understand and improve practice situations.

In an interview, one dietitian mentioned the ability to delve deeper into a situation—that is, the ability to ask, "What is going on? What's really happening here?"—as a key aspect of scientific inquiry. This questioning approach frequently resulted in dietitians uncovering previously overlooked, but crucial, information. For example, several dietitians mentioned discovering inappropriate insulin doses as a cause of underweight or overweight in patients. Another ruled out protein intake as a cause of persistently elevated blood urea nitrogen (BUN) level and worked with the medical and nursing team members in her setting to identify recirculating dialysis access. In each of these cases, the advanced practice dietitian identified problems that others had overlooked, and then used the information to improve practice patterns or develop more effective policies or procedures.

Techniques of Scientific Inquiry

In the context of advanced practice, "inquiry" is an umbrella term for the various activities used to organize and address the questions that a dietitian encounters in practice. For example, advanced practice dietitians use seemingly informal inquiry methods to elicit nutrition history and physical information, yet proceed from the general to the specific, pursuing productive lines of information and eliciting further information as needed. They rely on diagnostic reasoning to establish a nutrition diagnosis and select the most appropriate evidence-based intervention. Advanced practice dietitians are also involved in more formal investigations when they develop carefully designed research projects. This section discusses these three techniques of scientific inquiry, beginning with the scientific method, and then moving to diagnostic reasoning and evidence-based practice.

The Scientific Method

The true origin of scientific inquiry may never be known, although the Greek philosopher Socrates is often credited with developing this organized, questioning approach. The Socratic method, which is still used today, involves first proposing a hypothesis about a specific phenomenon and then examining this hypothesis by raising a series of questions in an effort to expose possible contradictions or inconsistencies. Generally, questioning continues until the hypothesis is either accepted or withdrawn. Socratic skills are highly regarded among medical professionals because they are academically challenging to develop. Such skills are applied in problem solving, in diagnostic reasoning, and in evidence-based practice.

The Socratic method is used to solve complex, evolving, or ambiguous problems. Medical and law school faculty members, for example, use this technique to stimulate critical analysis of complex and challenging legal or medical cases. In the typical application of the Socratic method, a case is presented and practitioners lead the presenter through a series of questions designed to prompt systematic consideration of alternative hypotheses or arguments. Eventually, the group agrees upon an acceptable argument, hypothesis, diagnosis, or intervention. Thus the Socratic method is a vehicle used to analyze a given situation, consider the possibilities, and derive a clear argument supporting the desired outcome.[4]

Although the Socratic method is an important teaching and reasoning strategy, it is also the foundation for the scientific method, which is widely taught and applied in medicine and dietetics. The scientific method is typically described as having four steps:

1. Observation and description of a phenomenon or a group of phenomena
2. Formulation of a hypothesis to explain the phenomenon
3. Use of the hypothesis to predict other phenomena
4. Testing of the experimental hypothesis

The scientific method is the basis of the research that drives clinical practice. The advanced practice dietitian may apply it to solve clinical problems, to develop a guideline or protocol, or to design a clinical research project. A more recent application of the scientific method is its incorporation into the diagnostic reasoning process.

Diagnostic Reasoning

The Nutrition Care Process is a four step problem solving method used by dietitians to identify a diagnosis which drives nutrition intervention, nutrition monitoring, and nutrition evaluation. When it was accepted by the dietetics profession in 2003, dietitians began to think carefully about nutrition diagnosis. When asked to see a patient, dietitians have tended to select an intervention based on items in the patient's nutrition history and physical examination. Some experienced diagnosticians and thought leaders, however, have looked to other fields for help in diagnostic reasoning. In medicine, the diagnostic process is well studied—a reflection of the high risk resulting from an incorrect or missed diagnosis. Thus numerous studies describe diagnostic reasoning strategies and identify how they differ from the novice to experienced diagnostician.[5]

Diagnostic reasoning strategies have been studied in medicine and nursing, and the research in these areas indicates that specific patterns emerge as expertise deepens. Elstein and Schwartz described the diagnostic reasoning of novices as a process of sequential hypothesis testing.[6] Using this model, the novice diagnostician solves difficult problems by first generating hypotheses and then systematically comparing them with sets of signs and symptoms. Additional tests are ordered to confirm or reject diagnoses until the correct diagnosis is established. This process, which is called hypothetico-deductive reasoning, parallels the scientific method. Although it is often used by novice practitioners who are learning the diagnostic process, it is time-consuming and requires extensive testing. The hypothetico-deductive method requires thorough data collection, but does not preclude ignoring or misinterpreting findings.

As practitioners gain more experience, their diagnostic reasoning process tends to depart from a strict, step-by-step application of the scientific approach. At the expert level, diagnostic reasoning is based less on a specific strategy and more on mastery of content.[6] Early in the diagnostic process, the expert develops a diagnosis, which is then confirmed by eliciting specific information from the patient (e.g., signs and symptoms, clinical history, and physical examination data). This strategy, which is called pattern recognition, is based on extensive accumulated experience with a repertoire of problems. Coderre and others describe pattern recognition as a complex mental process requiring rapid retrieval of an appropriate match for the diagnosis based on salient clues.[7] Because it relies on extensive experience, pattern recognition is generally unavailable to the novice.[7] According to Bloch and others, pattern recognition is a more perceptual, unconscious, probabilistic, and intuitive approach.[8] It enables rapid identification of the diagnosis, which is consistent with an advanced practice model. This approach enables the expert to identify a diagnosis both quickly and accurately. However, as Elstein and Schwartz observed, expert diagnosticians are not limited to scheme-based reasoning or pattern recognition alone, but rather revert to the hypothetico-deductive model when confronted with a new or difficult problem.[6]

The dietetics profession is just beginning to implement a formal scheme for diagnostic reasoning, so the processes used by dietitians to establish a diagnosis have not been thoroughly studied. Nevertheless, some of the elements of the hypothetico-deductive reasoning process are evident among dietitians who insist on obtaining laboratory data before completing a nutritional assessment. Informal observations reveal that more-experienced dietitians will often use fewer laboratory data to establish a diagnosis, ordering labs or tests only when the diagnosis is unclear. The nutrition care planning process, a complex process based on the identified problem or nutrition diagnosis, has been studied by Gates et al.[9,10] In these studies, the researchers found that novices were efficient in gathering data, but had more difficulty in formulating a nutrition care plan. Dietitians with a mean of seven years experience performed nutrition care planning significantly better than dietitians with less experience, suggesting that the outcomes obtained by novice and experienced dietitians differ as well.[9,10] Exhibit 5–1 highlights some of the experience-related differences in diagnostic reasoning for dietitians.

The nutrition diagnostic skills of dietitians will certainly be illuminated over time. Eventually, studies of diagnostic reasoning among dietitians will provide new insights into this process and opportunities to improve teaching and learning.

EXHIBIT 5–1

A Difference in Diagnostic Reasoning Between Novice and Expert Dietitians

The basic level RD will identify a patient with diabetes and an elevated hemoglobin A_{1c} level and provide diet instruction after obtaining a minimal nutrition history. The basic level dietitian uses the following thinking: Because the laboratory data are objective, they clearly identify a problem in nutrient intake. The novice dietitian presumes a knowledge deficit on the part of the patient and provides education on a diabetic diet.

The advanced practice dietitian will review the same data and ask the patient three or four targeted questions related to his or her usual food intake. From the answers, the advanced practice dietitian will discern that the patient has shifted his or her eating pattern based on a change in lifestyle, and will work with the patient on appropriate lifestyle modifications.

In the first situation, the patient is frustrated because he or she has heard this all before and tried to do it, but it isn't helping. The dietitian is frustrated because he or she is having to do the same thing all over again and perceives that the patient is not willing to adhere to the prescribed food and nutrition intervention. In the second situation, the patient is more amenable to the dietitian's suggestions because the intervention is targeted to the actual problem, and the advanced practice dietitian is more satisfied, because he or she has given the patient some useful information and will be able to measure progress on the next visit because both practitioner and patient have agreed on treating a specific issue with a specific therapy.

Evidence-Based Practice

For years, dietitians have taken a pragmatic approach toward MNT, accepting any practice that seems effective. As a result, clinical dietitians are taught and routinely use practices that are not well supported in the scientific literature. As the interest in cost-effective nutrition care has grown, and as the cry for positive outcomes that demonstrate value has become louder, evidence-based practice has emerged as a major issue throughout medicine in general and in MNT in particular. Evidence-based practice has been defined as the conscientious, explicit, and judicious use of current best evidence in making decisions about the care of individual patients.[11] It incorporates both clinical expertise and the best available external evidence from systematic research.

In dietetics, evidence-based practice is being developed based on a systematic and rigorous process.[12,13] Advanced practice dietitians and researchers have formulated practice questions, retrieved the relevant articles from the literature, and overseen grading of the literature for quality. Once the analysis is complete, findings are stated in a format that can be used by clinicians in practice. An example of an evidence-based statement appears in Table 5–1. Evidence analysis has also been used to develop guidelines for practice, which dietitians can then use to collect data demonstrating effective interventions.

Scientific Inquiry: A Summary

Evidence-based medicine does not result in a "cookbook" for nutrition intervention, nor does it replace clinical judgment. The skills of the advanced practice dietitian are still needed to apply both the evidence and the chosen interventions to achieve the desired results. The advanced practice dietitian applies evidence according to its meaning in the clinical realm, using clinical judgment in weighing alternative management strategies. In situations where evidence-based guidelines

---

Table 5–1 Example of an Evidence-Based Statement

Adult Weight Management Guideline
R.3 Optimal Length of Weight Management Therapy
R.3.0. Medical Nutrition Therapy for weight loss should last at least 6 months or until weight loss goals are achieved, with implementation of a weight maintenance program after that time. A greater frequency of contacts between the patient and practitioner may lead to more successful weight loss and maintenance. **Strong, Imperative**

Source: American Dietetic Association. Adult Weight Management Evidence Based Practice Guideline Available at http://www.adaevidencelibrary.com/topic.cfm?cat=3014. Accessed August 5, 2007.

are not yet available, the advanced practice dietitian reviews the existing evidence and ranks its value based on the strength of the evidence.

CREATIVITY

"It is the tension between creativity and skepticism that has produced the stunning and unexpected findings of science." —Carl Sagan[14]

Creativity has been defined as the power to create or, more appropriately for this discussion, as "having the quality of something created rather than imitated."[2] The word "creativity" typically conjures up a vision of an artist, sculptor, musician, or writer. In truth, creativity extends to the generation of ideas, practices, or things and hence is found across all disciplines. Creativity may also refer to connecting and rearranging knowledge. Funded researchers in the hard sciences, for example, speak of the need for creativity in approaching research problems. Likewise, business people highlight the role of creativity in sales, marketing, and product innovation. For their part, hospital administrators often urge creativity in dealing with the staffing and funding shortages that invariably plague those institutions. So, too, do advanced practice dietitians use creativity in their work.

The advanced practice dietitians interviewed for our study used creativity to innovate and to survive. Interviewees looked for—and found—inspiration everywhere. They stimulated their creativity with knowledge from other areas of dietetics, as well as from fields such as education, psychology, information science, medicine, and business. One suggested, "Once you get all these different ideas, you can integrate them and try to come up with creative solutions." Several interviewees mentioned thriving on change. Indeed, one defined advanced practice as "doing more than what we've always done." More than one advanced practice dietitian mentioned leaving a job when creativity was no longer possible. Exhibit 5–2 presents the use of creativity by one such advanced practice dietitian.

The concept of creativity is foreign to other dietitians, who view themselves as scientific rather than creative thinkers. These dietitians regard creativity as being inconsistent with the serious, science-based image of a medical nutrition therapist. Yet even in the most rigid of settings, managers frequently urge employees to "think outside the box" or use other creative techniques to overcome challenges. Creative programs designed to solve healthcare problems have been presented in quality management, health and safety, and healthcare redesign, for example.[15]

EXHIBIT 5–2

Using a Creative Approach

Where we are, there is no training for dietetic technicians, so we have to do it ourselves. At one point there was a real need for training, but there was really nothing available, so I got my staff together and we developed a training manual for technicians. At first I just used it for our facility, but other people began to talk about the problem of training techs: How did we do it and such?

At about the same time, I wanted to learn more about evidence analysis. We had tried to do some evidence analysis projects, and I needed better information. At that time, the best training was at the Cochrane Center in the United Kingdom. It was expensive to go there, but I needed the training.

I went to my boss and said, "I think we can market the diet tech training program. I want to try to sell it." Of course, I was scared. What if it didn't sell? But I told her that I thought I could sell five. Eventually we sold 30 of them, and I was able to use the money to get training at the Cochrane Center.

Structured approaches to creative thinking are available to help those who want to develop more creativity. For instance, Edward deBono's book *Six Thinking Hats* is widely used to solve problems in business and industry.[16] This approach can easily be applied to problems in health care and dietetics. Another resource is the work of Plsek, an engineer with a quality background who specializes in healthcare redesign. His principles for innovative thinking (listed in Table 5–2) can also be used to stimulate creativity.[15] These structured approaches to creativity are in line with the scientific thought process and may be comfortable for dietitians.

Creativity: A Summary

Creativity in the traditional artistic sense may not seem to fit within the scientific framework. However, a creative approach to common clinical situations may be an asset to advanced practice dietitians. Creativity may be used to solve complex scientific or patient related problems. Creativity may be developed using a structured approach to problems.

Table 5–2 Basic Heuristic Principles for Innovative Thinking

· Make it a habit to purposefully pause and notice things.
· Focus your creative energies on just a few topic areas that you genuinely care about and work on these areas purposefully for several weeks or months.
· Avoid being too narrow in the way you define your problem or topic area; try to use broader definitions, and see what insights you gain.
· Try to come up with original and useful ideas by making novel associations among things that you already know.
· When you need creative ideas, remember attention, escape, and movement.
· Pause and carefully examine ideas that make you laugh the first time you hear them.
· Recognize that your streams of thought and patterns of judgment are not inherently right or wrong; they are just what you think now, based primarily on patterns of your past.
· Make a deliberate effort to harvest, develop, and implement at least a few of the ideas you generate.

Source: Plsek P. Innovative thinking for the improvement of medical systems. *Annals of Internal Medicine* 1999;131(6):438–444.

BREADTH AND BALANCE OF PERSPECTIVE

"The test of a first-rate intelligence is the ability to hold two opposed ideas in mind at the same time and still retain the ability to function." —F. Scott Fitzgerald[17]

Breadth has been defined as something full of width, whereas balance is the stability produced by even distribution of weight on each side of a vertical axis.[2] These two concepts are not opposed to each other, but rather are somewhat related. Breadth is an important characteristic in drawing a distinction between advanced and specialty practice. It is the opposite of depth, which is the distinguishing descriptor of specialty knowledge and practice. Specialty practice focuses on every detail of a specific and often narrow topic. By contrast, advanced practice may be grounded in a specialty but sacrifices some detail to incorporate a broader range of knowledge. Incorporation of a broader perspective begets a balanced perspective.

In the study of advanced practice dietitians, the necessity of a broad perspective was expressed at the professional level as "connecting with other people's sciences and languages in order to provide a total treatment approach." At the patient level, breadth of perspective included understanding the whole picture, not just the nutritional issues. One interviewee spoke of the importance of "identifying the presence of co-morbidities and how they interface with medical nutrition therapy."

Another described looking beyond the nutrition component to the entire disease process and discerning that a diabetic patient was underweight because he was receiving insufficient insulin to achieve adequate glucose control. The result of both breadth and depth of perspective was thought to "get more at treating the total person. It's a more accurate way to plan treatment of an individual [who is] before you."

According to another interviewee,

> I felt it very refreshing to study in another area to broaden my understanding of practice. I was thinking if I did a Ph.D., I might even like to do that in psychology, because there is a lot to do in the psychology of eating, health behavior change, adopting healthy eating habits—those kinds of things. I find sometimes that I learn the most studying outside of the traditional areas of dietetic learning. Just because it's something new and fresh, I have to learn new terms but a different way of looking at things, problems, and problem solving.

Exhibit 5–3 provides an exemplar of the broader perspective espoused by one advanced practice dietitian.

EXHIBIT 5–3

A Broader Perspective

The specialist level dietitian was ready to discharge a patient on home enteral feedings. She had quickly and carefully calculated the formula and fluid prescription to meet the patient's needs and selected a specialized formula based on her knowledge from the literature on the topic. She knew the details of how to operate the feeding pump, and had investigated the pumps available from the homecare company so that the patient could be taught in the hospital exactly what to do at home. She had developed a set of orders and a schedule to change the patient to nighttime feedings according to a policy in place in her department. She had called the homecare company and ordered the formula and equipment. The transfer orders were ready for the physician signature.

On rounds, the physician asked the patient if he was ready to go home, and the patient replied, "Yes." The dietitian explained that the patient would be going home on nighttime feedings over 12 hours from 8 P.M. to 8 A.M., when

continues

EXHIBIT 5–3 *continued*

the patient quietly but emphatically interjected, "No! I have something else to do at night."

In the same situation, the advanced practice RD began the process by talking with the patient about tube feedings and what was involved in giving them at home. During the interview, the patient revealed that he worked the night shift at a sheet metal fabrication plant. The dietitian explained that several different scheduling options were available and asked when the patient thought it would be better to do the feedings—daytime, nighttime, or possibly a split schedule. Before she specified a formula, she checked with the discharge planner to identify what type of coverage was available to assist the patient with the costs. Then she developed a feeding plan that utilized available resources, including the local drugstore, which would deliver items to the patient's home.

By soliciting this information and engaging the patient in the process, time was saved in tailoring the plan to the patient. Ideally, giving the patient some control over the situation would improve compliance as well.

Breadth and balance require having a shared perspective with others—that is, identifying how the nutrition intervention fits into the total treatment plan. The advanced practice dietitian is able to ask whether a specific therapy is a primary necessity in treating the overall patient, just a detail, or a "nice but not necessary" part of the plan. The advanced practice dietitian is also able to see things from the patient's perspective, including issues of food and culture, the patient's viewpoint on health and disease, and food and nutrients. In regard to balance, one dietitian said, "A really effective person needs to be able to pull in the necessary details to solve the big picture, share the problem, or go wherever you are working toward, yet be able to move back and forth between the two extremes of clinical dietetics."

Breadth and Balance: A Summary

Depth of knowledge in a particular area is often a goal for dietitians. However, breadth and balance of knowledge is likely a defining characteristic of the advanced practice dietitian. While advanced practice dietitians are often experts in a specific area of practice, it is the breadth of the approach and the ability to balance the different facets of a situation that distinguish advanced practice.

SUMMARY

Three components of the attitude sub-theme—scientific inquiry, creativity, and breadth and balance of perspective—begin to distinguish advanced practice dietitians from specialists, generalists, and basic level practitioners. These skills can be learned and developed through directed reading, through coursework, and with the aid of mentoring from teachers and colleagues.

KEY POINTS

- The advanced practice dietitian looks beyond the surface of a situation, delves more deeply into it, and asks why or why not. He or she searches to find answers to questions using rational thinking, available evidence, and accepted methods of scientific inquiry.
- The advanced practice dietitian provides a creative perspective based on a wealth of practice experience and information. He or she may not be creative in the artistic sense, but has developed the ability to apply a creative approach to practice.
- The advanced practice dietitian differs from specialist dietitians in being able to draw upon a wealth of information from other disciplines and apply it to problems in medical nutrition therapy. The breadth of information that distinguishes advanced practice is the opposite of the depth of information that characterizes specialty practice.

SUGGESTED READING

Scientific Inquiry

American Dietetic Association. Evidence analysis library. Available at http://www.adaevidence library.com/default.cfm?library=EAL.

> This growing library contains hundreds of dietetics-related papers that have been reviewed according to stringent criteria by trained evidence analysts. For some topics, evidence-based guidelines are already available; more are under development.

Bowen JL. Educational strategies to promote clinical diagnostic reasoning. *New England Journal of Medicine* 2006;355:2217–2225.

The Cochrane collection. Available at http://www.cochrane.org/index.htm.

This British-based international organization performs evidence-based reviews of topics of interest in medicine. Its website offers a number of nutrition-related reviews concerning infant and neonatal nutrition, early enteral feeding in patients with a variety of medical conditions, and wounds.

The CONSORT statement. Available at http://www.consort-statement.org.

This website contains documents with extensive recommendations from a group of researchers, editors, and statisticians concerning the correct reporting of clinical trials.

The Socratic method. Available at http://www.law.uchicago.edu/socrates/soc_article.html.

This article is adapted from one published in *The Green Bag* by Elizabeth Garrett in 1998. It explains the basics of the Socratic method.

Creativity

American Creativity Association. Available at http://www.amcreativityassoc.org/index.htm.

The American Creativity Association website provides sample exercises, information, reference materials, and ideas. There is an extensive bibliography in case you're really into this topic.

Csikszentmihalyi M. *Creativity*. New York: Harper Collins, 1996.

A classic study of creativity for those with an academic bent.

deBono E. *Six thinking hats*. London: Penguin Books, 1999.

This brief and easy-to-read book provides six ways of thinking about issues. One strategy is a structured approach to creativity, which may be useful to those with a scientific mindset.

Directed Creativity. Available at http://www.directedcreativity.com/.

Creativity for serious people is available from Directed Creativity, the website of Paul E. Plsek. This site is a comfortable fit for those with a scientific mindset. It contains models and tools for creativity. The author lists a number of works related to healthcare quality, and his working paper titled "Models for the Creative Process" provides a quick overview of models for creative change.

Johnson S. *Who moved my cheese?* New York: G. P. Putnam's Sons, 1998.

A fable about adapting to change.

MacKinzie G. *Orbiting the giant hairball*. Shawnee Mission, KS: OpusPocus, 1996.

A quick read and a clever book about how a creative person survived and thrived in corporate America.

Mycoted. Available at http://www.mycoted.com/creativity/techniques/index.php; http://www.mycoted.com/Main_Page.

A nice introduction to creativity may be found on the website operated by Mycoted, a small British consulting firm. Its website lists creativity techniques along with brief explanations of their use.

Breadth and Balance of Perspective

Fadiman A. *The spirit catches you and you fall down*. New York: Farrar, Strauss and Giroux, 1997.

This book clearly illustrates problems in healthcare communication.

Gordon S. *Nursing against the odds*. Ithaca, NY: Cornell University Press, 2005.

> This text highlights major issues not just in nursing but also in health care in general. It explains much about the relationships between physicians, nurses, and other professionals.

Shilts R. *And the band played on*. New York: St. Martin's Press, 1987.

> This readable book provides insight into U.S. health policy, epidemiology, and the perspective of patients with AIDS.

Starr P. *The social transformation of American medicine*. New York: Basic, 1982.

> This classic academic volume provides insight into our current medical structure.

EXPERIENCES TO TRY

Scientific Inquiry

1. Go to guidelines.gov and enter "nutrition" as a search term. Are there guidelines that apply to your practice? Print one or two of them out, then repeat the same exercise with the Cochrane Collection and the ADA's evidence analysis library. What are the topics covered? Are there differences in how the guidelines are stated? Look carefully to determine whether there are differences in the level of rigor applied to the data analysis supporting the recommendations.

2. To develop a better understanding of evidence-based practice in dietetics, go to the ADA's evidence analysis library. Access some of the evidence-based guidelines and familiarize yourself with the grades assigned to the recommendations. Review the questions and the evidence summaries supporting the recommendations. Finally, review some of the original articles and the analysts' recommendations.

3. Select a recurring problem common to your patient population. Locate several articles that would apply to this problem. Look the articles over, rank them according to their quality, and then apply the ADA's quality guidelines to them. Does your analysis differ based on applying the same, objective criteria?

Creativity

1. Download and work through some of the exercises on the websites listed in the Suggested Reading section.

2. Attend an educational session, lecture, or symposium on a topic that is new to you. Afterward, take a few minutes and jot down notes about how you think you could use or relate the information to your practice.

3. Join an organization that is "outside your box." Read its newsletter for a year, and then evaluate how the information influenced your own practice.

4. Identify a problem that you would like to solve creatively. Apply the heuristic in Table 5–1 and think through the problem with a colleague. Are you able to come up with something different?

Breadth and Balance of Perspective

1. Go to your favorite library or bookstore. Identify a book that would provide insight into a particular patient population. Obtain and read it. Try to read one such book each year.

2. Go to a medical library and locate standard introductory texts for medicine, surgery, nursing, pharmacy, physical therapy, social work, and dietetics. Locate the chapter in each book that introduces the student to the profession. Read these chapters and make a list of the main points of each chapter. Compare the main points across professions. Are they similar? Different? To which profession is dietetics most similar? Most dissimilar? Based on your experience in dietetics, how could the dietetics chapter be improved?

3. Sign up to receive the free online table of contents of two or three journals that you don't normally read. Read each table of contents and see what catches your eye. Make a list of these items. At the end of a year, look over this list and see if your perspective has broadened.

4. Pretend to be a patient with a newly diagnosed disease and try to find information on your condition. "Google" the disease and see what comes up. Go to the website operated by the foundation for the disease, the National Institutes of Health (NIH) website, and a patient support site, and compare the general and nutrition information that is available from these sources. Go to bookstore, and see what is available there. Go to a health food store and impersonate someone with the disease. Interview other health professionals to get their perspective on how they approach this type of patient. Keep notes on the different perspectives that you identify, and compare them.

5. Go to Pub Med and enter a topic of interest to you. Select two or three articles, and then follow the links for the names of the authors. Pay attention to the breadth of topics they write about.

REFERENCES

1. Williams E. Available at http://www.wisdomquotes.com/002629.html. Accessed April 17, 2007.
2. Merriam-Webster Online. Available at www.m-w.com/. Accessed July 5, 2006.
3. Thinkexist.com. Available at http://thinkexist.com/quotation/there_are_two_ways_to_slide_easily_through_life/12677.html. Accessed February 7, 2007.
4. Bowen JL. Educational strategies to promote clinical diagnostic reasoning. *New England Journal of Medicine* 2006;355(21):2217–2225.
5. Patel VL, Kaufman DR, Arocha JF. Emerging paradigms of cognition in medical decision-making. *Journal of Biomedical Informatics* 2002;35(1):52–75.
6. Elstein AS, Schwarz A. Clinical problem solving and diagnostic decision making: Selective review of the cognitive literature. *British Medical Journal* 2002;324(7339): 729–732.
7. Coderre S, Mandin H, Harasym PH, Fick GH. Diagnostic reasoning strategies and diagnostic success. *Medical Education* 2003;37(8):695–703.
8. Bloch RL, Hofer D, Feller S, Hodel M. The role of strategy and redundancy in diagnostic reasoning. *BMC Medical Education* 2003;3:1–12.
9. Gates GE, Kris-Etherton PM, Greene G. Nutrition care planning: Comparison of the skills of dietitians, interns, and students. *Journal of the American Dietetic Association* 1990;90(10):1393–1397.
10. Gates GE, Meyer GR. Dietitians' disease-specific nutrition care planning strategies. *Journal of the American Dietetic Association* 1994;94(1):81–83.
11. Sackett DL, Richardson WS, Rosenberg W, Haynes RB. *Evidence-based medicine; How to practice and teach EBM.* Edinburgh: Churchill Livingstone, 1998.
12. American Dietetic Association. Evidence analysis library. Available at http://www.adaevidencelibrary.com/default.cfm?auth=1. Accessed April 17, 2007.
13. American Dietetic Association. *ADA Evidence Analysis Manual.* Chicago: American Dietetic Association, 2005.
14. Wisdom quotes. Available at http://www.wisdomquotes.com/002629.html. Accessed April 17, 2007.
15. Plsek P. Innovative thinking for the improvement of medical systems. *Annals of Internal Medicine* 1999;131(6):438–444.
16. deBono E. *Six thinking hats.* London: Penguin Books, 1999.
17. Brainy quote. Available at http://www.brainyquote.com/. Accessed March 13, 2007.

Context

Summary

Key Points

Suggested Reading

Experiences to Try

References

"Always design a thing by considering it in its next larger context—a chair in a room, a room in a house, a house in an environment, an environment in a city plan."
—Eliel Saarinen[1]

The context sub-theme of the advanced practice model refers to the dynamic relationship between the advanced practice dietitian and the professional environment. Along the path to advanced practice, the dietitian focuses less on developing additional technical knowledge needed for specialty practice and begins to develop contextual skills. The advanced practice dietitian retains expertise in direct clinical practice, but has developed and incorporated expanded contextual skills to augment his or her effectiveness. The result is that the advanced practice dietitian understands and is influenced by contextual factors in the environment and, conversely, exerts influence on those same factors.

The practice context is shaped by a number of factors, including the setting; the geographic location; the patient population served; legal, regulatory, and economic constraints; and institutional and professional roles and traditions. Within the practice context are several sub-themes used by advanced practice dietitians to define and expand the nature and scope of services provided. Using collaboration, networking, consultation, leadership, and awareness, the advanced practice dietitian in medical nutrition therapy influences both patients (either alone or in groups) and the environment of practice. This chapter provides background and examples of the advanced practice context.

COLLABORATION

"None of us are as smart as all of us." —Japanese proverb[2]

Collaboration is defined as working "jointly with others or together especially in an intellectual endeavor."[3] As health care has become more complex, more specialized, and more fragmented, collaboration between caregivers has been increasingly recognized as an important aspect of practice. It is used to increase diagnostic and problem-solving capacity and to provide complex and comprehensive care. Collaboration between health professionals is currently being promoted because the exchange of information between caregivers offers a means to improve healthcare quality and safety.[4] According to Nugent and Lambert, collaborative practice is based on professionals functioning as colleagues and partners within a "flat hierarchy" rather than within the traditional vertically structured, physician-dominated model.[5] In a collaborative environment, the members of each profession involved contribute their expertise to the total plan of care for the patient and share that plan of care with other caregivers.

Two terms may be used to help distinguish between basic and advanced level practice with respect to collaboration: multidisciplinary and interdisciplinary.

- *Multidisciplinary* care is the sequential provision of disciplinary specific health care by multiple providers.[6]
- *Interdisciplinary* collaborative care is a process of coordination, joint decision making, and communication with shared responsibility and shared authority.[6]

Dietitians function in either a multidisciplinary or interdisciplinary role. In a multidisciplinary environment, the registered dietitian functions alone without considering the total plan for patient care or the way in which the nutrition care plan affects the work of other disciplines. This description is typical of basic level dietetics practice. By contrast, the interdisciplinary practitioner works to form a cohesive plan, developed in collaboration with others, and assumes shared responsibility for care that results in shared authority. Because it requires more expertise, more confidence, and a greater breadth of knowledge, the interdisciplinary approach is consistent with advanced practice.

Collaboration in Advanced Dietetics Practice

In the study conducted by this book's authors, advanced practice dietitians described collaboration as the need to be connected through teamwork with other individuals.[7] Indeed, they viewed understanding the roles and perspectives of nurses, physicians, pharmacists, and others involved in patient care as an essential skill. When asked to describe the difference in basic and advanced level practice, one advanced practice dietitian defined the basic level practitioner as someone who sits next to another health professional but remains within the dietetics silo, whereas the advanced level practitioner actively works together with a variety of other practitioners. This illustration supports the interdisciplinary and multidisciplinary distinction between basic and advanced practice.

Advanced practice dietitians consider the interdisciplinary team or approach to be a viable means to enhance patient care. One dietitian described the necessity of being "where the decisions are made" as a means of efficiently managing patient care. Another described reviewing the services she typically provided with new referring physicians. After they were made aware of the services she could provide, she asked physicians to select the ones they would prefer she deliver to their patients. Advanced practice dietitians also described groups of colleagues who formed teams, committees, or task forces to develop collaborative protocols, solve patient care problems, or develop process improvement projects.

The advanced practice dietitians in our study collaborated with numerous other professionals, including those from medicine and surgery, pharmacy, nursing, social work, speech therapy, physical therapy, and occupational therapy. They also collaborated with patients and families to achieve the desired results. For many of the dietitians in our study, a collaborative environment resulted in expanding or crossing traditional role boundaries. Several dietitians described functioning interchangeably with the pharmacist or nurse in providing medication or wound care information. These advanced practice dietitians also taught other team members basic nutrition information so as to ensure that patients received consistent information. They found that teaching basic nutrition information to physicians, nurses, and others enabled them to focus on higher-level nutrition activities.

Collaboration in Health Care

Collaborative practice is increasingly being advocated by bodies such as the Institute of Medicine, which recommends that all health professionals be trained in interdisciplinary collaboration.[8] Similarly, the Joint Commission (formerly the Joint Commission on Accreditation of Healthcare Organizations) requests demonstration of interdisciplinary care as part of the accreditation process.[9] Successful collaboration requires time—a precious commodity that is in short supply in many institutions. Collaborative time is not well reimbursed, so that it is necessary to document cost and error reductions that result from collaboration. The results of collaboration between health professionals are being measured, and their positive impact on safety and costs have been documented. For example, collaboration between pharmacists and physicians during patient care rounds in an intensive care unit has been shown to reduce adverse drug events, heart failure, and costs.[10–12] Collaboration between disciplines may also decrease length of stay in trauma units.[13] In an office-based practice, interdisciplinary collaboration between social workers, nurses, and physicians reduced healthcare utilization even as it maintained the health status of patients.[14]

Collaboration is enhanced when professionals attending rounds together develop an understanding of each other's professional roles, skills, and philosophy.[6] It is also enhanced when there is recognition and respect for the educational background and expertise of other professionals.[6] Because the education and training of health professionals are not always well understood, advanced practice dietitians may need to educate themselves about the level of training required for jobs in other health professions. They may also take advantage of opportunities to explain the educational background and special skills of the dietitian.

Collaboration is enhanced in an environment where information, power, and authority are shared. Likewise, it is enhanced by the confidence in one's knowledge and skills that come with experience. **Table 6–1** lists some of the collaborative skills that are key to advanced practice dietitians.

Table 6–1 Collaboration Skills

- Focus on the patient problem and how it might be improved. State goals for intervention from the patient's perspective rather than from the caregiver's perspective.
- Learn to speak the language of collaboration—for example, using "we" rather than "I." Avoid discipline-specific jargon.
- Negotiate your role in advance, but only after understanding your skills and scope of practice, and the skills and scope of practice of others.
- Reflect regularly on your own contribution and ways to use your skills to fulfill unmet needs within the group.
- Be open to new ideas and welcoming of input from others while sharing information and resources.
- Contribute to a positive environment by avoiding criticism of others.
- Perfect your conflict resolution skills.
- Thank people for their contributions.
- Always maintain a sense of humor.

To date, the collaborative activities of dietitians have not been well described in the literature. Nevertheless, it is known that dietitians collaborate with nephrologists and nurses in dialysis centers, with surgeons and gastroenterologists on nutrition support teams, and with intensivists in burn and critical care units. (See **Exhibit 6–1** for an example related to MNT for renal patients.) Several of the dietitians interviewed for our study collaborated with endocrinologists and nurses in diabetes practice. In fact, current regulations mandate dietitian participation in oversight of diabetes self-management programs.[15] In some situations, the details of collaboration are specified in policies, procedures, or legal contracts, such as collaborative practice agreements, but few data are available to illuminate the collaboration skills of dietitians.

EXHIBIT 6–1

Using Roundsmanship to Enhance Collaborative Practice

When I came here, a standard "no potassium, no protein" diet was ordered for most renal patients. This practice created confusion and disrupted continuity of care for chronic dialysis patients, who were educated to a more liberal approach. My written recommendations to liberalize diets seemed futile, as busy physicians focused on more critical and time-sensitive problems than diet order. I quickly learned that decisions were made during interdisciplinary rounds with nurses, residents, pharmacists, and the social worker. If I was to be effective, I would have to present my plan to the group during rounds. Of course, this activity would take time from an already busy day, but I was looking for a payoff in terms of reduced frustration both for my patients and for myself.

I noted the duration of rounds, and the amount of time I spent on the unit using the current system. For a couple of weeks, I monitored the fate of my recommendations, noting which were ignored and which were implemented. It was interesting to find that I spent about as much time trying to explain incorrect diet orders to patients and staff as they were spending in rounds. I discussed my findings with the clinical nutrition manager, who agreed to a new model of care as long as my other responsibilities were not neglected.

EXHIBIT 6–1 *continued*

I contacted the head nurse and the physician unit director to let them know that I would be attending rounds. To prepare for my participation, I spent an afternoon in the medical library reviewing key information on nutritional management of renal disease. I also scanned the table of contents from recent renal journals to make sure I was current with what physicians were reading.

On the appointed day, I arrived a half-hour before rounds and quickly identified the renal patients on the unit. I obtained data to estimate how well each patient was eating; I also wrote down the current diet order as well as the patient's most recent height and weight. There was no need to record other information as the resident presented lab results, medications, and other clinical data during rounds. I quickly compared the estimated oral intake to the estimated needs for each patient and then reviewed my notes regarding potential nutrition diagnoses, concerns raised by the nurse or patient, and the most likely nutrition intervention for each patient on the list.

I established mental priorities so that I could discuss the intervention that might have the greatest impact first. During the first presentation, I quickly observed that the attending was decisive and wanted only the most essential information, but seemed receptive to input from others. I adapted my comments accordingly, holding details in reserve until needed.

Soon, people began to ask questions related to MNT for renal disease. I offered to provide physicians and nurses with an in-service program on the Kidney Disease Outcomes Quality Initiative (K-DOQI) guidelines and some related literature. My offer was accepted. I prepared carefully, and the presentation was well received.

During the first month, I collected data documenting how much time I spent on the unit each day and developed a form where I recorded the patients seen, their nutrition diagnoses, interventions, and outcomes. I also collected information during my conversations with nurses about how much happier the patients were with their diets, and shared that information with the clinical nutrition manager. It took a few weeks to get things into shape on that unit, but attending rounds really helped me to work efficiently and quickly become a productive member of the team.

Collaboration: A Summary

Collaboration is a recommended skill for improving patient care. Dietitians who participate in interdisciplinary collaboration and shared decision making create more extensive opportunities to integrate nutrition into the overall plan of care. Collaborative practice enhances a comprehensive approach to the patient. Collaboration also enhances effective and efficient implementation of nutrition intervention. In particular, it provides opportunities for the advanced practice dietitian to demonstrate the contributions that MNT might make to the overall plan of care.

NETWORKING

"I not only use all the brains I have, but all that I can borrow." —*Woodrow Wilson*[16]

Networking has been used by people in all professions to exchange information or services among individuals, groups, or institutions.[3] Healthcare workers, for example, use networks to disseminate, obtain, or exchange information.[17] Professionals may also use networks to obtain work or to seek out new job and career opportunities. Some take advantage of networks to seek or provide mentoring. Others use networks to maintain their current knowledge or to implement changes in practice. Another use for networks is to foster collaborative research or practice projects.

Networking in Advanced Practice Dietetics

The advanced practice dietitians in our study participated in well-developed interprofessional networks. They exchanged information or developed intellectual partnerships with physicians, educators, administrators, nurses, and others. They also valued their networks with other dietitians. In fact, several dietitians who participated in our study cited networking opportunities as the primary reason to volunteer for professional activities.

One advanced practice dietitian used an extended network to multiply the ideas generated by her staff:

> The main thing is the external partnership, because we get so many e-mails that say, "Oh, I want to know more" or "Could we bring this further, if we work together?" . . . we may only have 7 bodies here, but with all these contacts, it is like

50 dietitians that are sort of connecting with us . . . to advance practice in different ways. I think we need to have more networking and getting out there.

For others, networking was viewed less as a means for advancing an agenda and more as a way to develop relationships with other, like-minded people: "Trying to get together and just talking ideas, just hearing what they're doing—that's where I really feel that I'm invigorated."

Advanced practice dietitians used electronic "list-servs" (list servers—essentially electronic bulletin boards) to participate in communities organized around a practice area, usually with a professional association acting as sponsor. Electronic networks have helped dietitians in remote locations participate and "meet" others. It is possible that some advanced practice dietitians have developed larger networks using this medium. While research on social networks suggests that the average person can maintain contact with approximately 150 persons, an electronic network or list-serv might potentially increase this number dramatically.[18] Some networks are used to conduct fairly high-level discussions. Others are used to obtain advice on difficult or unfamiliar situations or to share breaking news, as in the example in **Exhibit 6–2.** Occasionally, messages are circulated across networks to obtain broader input. Clearly, electronic networking has allowed dietitians to extend their networks to encompass greater numbers of people and to obtain a wider perspective on issues.

The literature on networking is sparse, especially among dietitians. Bradley et al. found that even before electronic networking was available, advanced practice dietitians had large networks of colleagues.[19] Skipper and Lewis found that advanced practice dietitians included physicians, nurses, and others in their networks.[7] In addition, advanced practice dietitians had contacts in their communities and through other organizations. Many knew senior policy officials in their organization, community, or legislature. Some advanced practice dietitians used practice or special-interest groups to obtain and share information. Others had established their own networks of colleagues.

Networking: A Summary

Advanced practice dietitians typically have well-developed networks of colleagues that span both disciplines and geographic areas. They use these networks as extra "hands" or extra "brains" to provide information and solve problems. These dietitians also contribute to such networks, thereby providing information to their colleagues.

EXHIBIT 6-2

Obtaining Information on Breaking News

On the way into work, I heard that a radio report on a *New England Journal of Medicine* article that implicated blue food coloring in the deaths of patients receiving tube feedings. Knowing this would be an issue as soon as I walked in the door at the hospital, I called my colleague, who was already at work in the Midwest. Sure enough, she was in her office, but she had not yet heard the news. Even so, in a few seconds, she pulled up the article in question on her computer and read it to me over the phone. I gave her my fax number, and the article was on my desk when I arrived in my office.

In the interim, my colleague called a former employee, who worked for one of the major enteral formula manufacturers, to get the company's read on the information. I called our pulmonologists to make them aware of the situation just as my colleague e-mailed me with a message from the formula manufacturer.

Both of us worked in our respective institutions to immediately remove the blue food coloring from the patient care areas in our hospitals, then shared information and strategies with each other and with colleagues around the country as the situation developed. In fact, my memo to nursing concerning the change to our policy was drafted with input from my colleagues around the country.

CONSULTATION

"I do not recommend every corpulent man to rush headlong into such a change of diet (certainly not), but to act advisedly and after full consultation with a physician."
—*William Banting*[16]

Consultation has been defined as a deliberation between physicians on a case or its treatment.[3] In the case of the advanced practice dietitian, this definition could be modified to "a deliberation between the dietitian and the physician, nurse practitioner, or physician assistant on a case or its treatment," as any of these primary care providers may request consultation services from the dietitian. Certainly the quote that introduces this section would be modified today to refer to dietitians. The reciprocal of consultation is a referral—that is, the act of sending a patient to another health professional (including another dietitian). The term "referral" may also apply to the actual document authorizing a visit to another health professional. The concepts of consultation and referral are closely related and will be discussed together in this section.

The consultation and referral process is a basic component of healthcare practice. It incorporates two principles:

1. A single individual—usually a physician or nurse practitioner—is the primary care provider for a patient. This individual maintains an ongoing relationship with the patient, treats the majority of medical problems, and coordinates care provided by others.
2. Medical care is complex, and a single individual does not possess all the skills needed to provide expert care in all situations.

In recognition of the second principle, the primary care provider refers complex or difficult patients to consultants, including advanced practice dietitians, for treatment of problems beyond their expertise or interest. To do so effectively, primary care providers seek and maintain a network of consultants to provide expert care for their patients. Consultants, in turn, seek a network of primary care providers that refer patients for treatment. In fact, the consultation–referral process is so ingrained in the healthcare system that a referral is required as a prerequisite for payment for MNT encounters.

Consultation versus Referral

Our study of advanced practice dietitians revealed that those working in outpatient settings used the consultation–referral model as a source of patients, learned to work with the existing reimbursement mechanisms, and obtained reimbursement for their services. The dietitians interviewed for this study functioned as independent practitioners, confident that their recommendations were valued and that they were making a positive contribution to both the patient and the team of caregivers. One dietitian mentioned consulting with other dietitians with expertise outside her area to obtain the best care for a patient. Another dietitian collaborated with physicians concerning insulin management and carbohydrate intake for patients with diabetes. These advanced practice dietitians derived satisfaction from seeking or providing consultation with other dietitians on difficult cases, or being asked to share their expertise by teaching students or clinicians from dietetics, medicine, pharmacy, nursing, or other disciplines.

The consultant role filled by the advanced practice dietitian differs from the duties that are performed in basic level practice. That is, the basic level dietitian in a hospital or long-term care facility "sees" patients based on the results of hospital-wide screening at admission. The basic level dietitian performs a nutrition assessment, writes recommendations in the medical record, and awaits those recommendations' implementation by physician order. A major disadvantage of this model is that it places dietitians in the unenviable position of providing unsolicited recommendations to physicians who have not requested their services. Not surprisingly, these unanticipated recommendations are sometimes ignored or—albeit rarely—greeted with hostility.

The consultation–referral process is not widely understood in dietetics. Nevertheless, it is widely used in health care and has been adopted by many advanced practice dietitians. The advanced practice dietitian typically sees patients who are referred for treatment of a specific nutrition problem; as a result, the dietitian usually restricts his or her practice to a few types of patients so as to maintain the necessary depth and breadth of expertise required to provide current, effective interventions for those problems. Implementation of this model means that the dietitian becomes comfortable with the idea that not every patient needs, wants, or would benefit from nutrition intervention. In addition, the successful consultant dietitian must become expert at documenting the results of the consultation and communicating the nutritional plan to the physician. The exemplar contains an example of a consultant's letter to a referring physician (**Exhibit 6–3**).

EXHIBIT 6–3

Consultation Letter for an Overweight Patient

August 30, 2007
Re: James Jones

Dear Dr. Ahern,

Thank you for asking me to assist in the care of your patient, James Jones who was seen in my office today (August 30, 2007) for an initial evaluation of diet in light of recent weight gain, which I believe results from an excess oral food and beverage intake related to a decline in his activity level

EXHIBIT 6–3 *continued*

compared to his food intake as evidenced by his diet and activity history. His height is 5'11" with a weight of 207# and a BMI of 28.9 which places him in the overweight category. I am concerned that his blood pressure was 149/92 mmHg when I measured it today. As you know, this is consistent with stage I hypertension. At this stage of his treatment, the issues which should be addressed include 1) establishing the primary cause of the changes in his weight and activity level, 2) jointly establishing realistic weight management goals, 3) initiating a counseling program that will support Mr. Jones in adopting healthier behaviors related to eating, activity and weight. I believe that he will benefit from intensive and individualized counseling for 12 weeks which will ultimately decrease his weight and in concert with medical management, his blood pressure.

My goal is to assist you in your patient's care, providing appropriate consultation and management of Mr. Jones' nutrition related issues. I anticipate that, over the next year, I will need to see him weekly for the first 12 weeks, then every three months. I would most appreciate if your office would arrange the following tests for him and forward them to my office by September 15th.

Fasting Blood Glucose
Lipid Profile including HDL and LDL cholesterol.

With your permission, the areas I would like to focus my attention in the care of your patient with overweight are:

1) Reduced overall intake of oral food and beverages with an agreed upon goal of sustainable weight loss 2) Gradual implementation of a DASH-type diet incorporating a decreased sodium intake 3) Increased physical activity level 4) Increased calcium and potassium intake with supplements based on usual intake.

If you would like to primarily manage any of the above areas of care, please let me know. We can then agree on appropriate goals. I will be sure that you get a letter or other form of communication from me after each office visit.

Sincerely yours,

Janice Heibert, DCN, RD

Table 6–2 The American Society of Family Practice Physicians' Definition of Consultation

---

1. The consultation is a request from a physician for an intervention or advisory opinion.
2. The patient should have a clear understanding of the consultation process and is free to offer suggestions.
3. The request for a consultation for patients should be documented in writing, and should be accompanied by relevant medical information.
4. The consultant performs a requested intervention and/or makes recommendations regarding diagnosis and/or treatment in a timely manner, but does not initiate other treatment. A written report of findings and recommendations should become part of the patient's record.
5. The patient remains in the care of the physician who requested the consultation.
6. The physician who requested the consultation uses professional judgment in deciding whether to act on the consultant's recommendation.
7. Other considerations (e.g., patient request, conflicting recommendations, medical or other concerns) may cause the physician who requested the consultation to seek another opinion.

Source: The American Academy of Family Physicians. Available at http://www.aafp.org/online/en/home/policy/policies/c/consultationdefinition.html. Accessed October 4, 2007.

Dietitian effectiveness using the models described previously has been studied. For example, Skipper et al. found that about 45% of dietitians' recommendations were implemented; dietitian effectiveness was improved to more than 65%, however, when a consultative model was used.[20] This finding is similar to the concordance rate for physician-to-physician consultation. A valuable perspective on the physician's viewpoint may be gained by reviewing the definition of consultation provided in **Table 6–2.** Although data on the topic are scarce, it is postulated that most referrals to a dietitian are for interventions such as education, counseling, or modification of MNT.

The Consultation–Referral Process: A Summary

A basic understanding of the consultation–referral process would reduce frustration for all dietitians practicing in acute care. The value of the consultant role is that it places the advanced practice dietitian on a higher level and creates a different relationship with other healthcare professionals. Even in situations where such services are not directly reimbursed, the act of consulting the advanced practice dietitian ensures that the service has greater intrinsic value because some effort is involved in obtaining the consultation. Also, for dietitians who work in outpatient or private practice settings, consultations are often their primary source of revenue.

LEADERSHIP

"Leadership is the ability to create followership." —*Joe Smith*

There are likely as many different definitions for leadership as there are authors on the subject. *Webster's Dictionary* defines leadership as the capacity to lead and further defines a leader as one who has commanding authority or influence.[3] Heifetz offers a definition that may be more practical for dietitians: He states that leaders prepare people for change.[21] Heifetz also provides examples of a single individual leading a family, a small group of individuals, a community, or an entire country.[2] His definition may be appropriate to dietitians who are in a position to lead change in the lives of their patients, their workplace, their profession, or their community.

Leadership is a relatively new topic for dietitians. It has been defined by the profession as the "ability to inspire and guide others toward building and achieving a shared vision."[22] Leadership skills will be useful for dietitians who are transitioning to an advanced practice role, and to help other practitioners adapt to the emergence of that role. Thus there is a clear need for advanced practice dietitians to obtain leadership skills.

The advanced practice dietitians that we interviewed were conscious of leadership activities, and were especially proud of their success in changing practice. One described leadership as the ability to make a contribution or to make a difference. Another advanced practice dietitian described being invited to a foreign country to change practice as an example of leadership. A third described leadership in her work setting as "the ability to build a team and then lead that team on nutritional issues." This dietitian had trained nurses to do some basic nutrition tasks and described herself as "leading" rather than always "doing" nutrition. One advanced practice dietitian described contacting officers of a national professional organization to facilitate a response to a federal agency concerning a nutrition-related issue in her area of practice. Another mentioned involvement with policy issues within professional organizations and government. All cited examples of participating as change agents in various paid or volunteer roles.

Advanced practice dietitians exhibit authority. They expect to be heard and to make a difference. They are confident and positive in their approach, seeking opportunities that reflect their ability to define a place for themselves. These professionals persevere in developing new programs and projects, and they prevail under adverse circumstances. They actively pursue both professional and work agendas, sometimes in the face of overwhelming odds.

One advanced practice dietitian described her ability to maintain her optimism in the face of serious threats to her job during a hospital reorganization. Another cited her ability to "weather the storm" by thinking broadly about her career during both personal and professional difficulties. These advanced practice dietitians described formal leadership roles in management, whether in elected or appointed positions. They also filled informal leadership roles as senior staff members or as members of committees or informal groups. Although all of these interviewees had been invited speakers and were authors in their specific area of practice, these accomplishments were mentioned in an offhand way. These activities were not considered a defining characteristic of leaders, but rather functioned as more of a prerequisite or vehicle for distributing information toward a desired end.

The Study of Leadership

Leadership is being incorporated into many professions as a means to help practitioners from all disciplines adapt to changes in the work environment. Managers, in particular, often attend leadership meetings and training. Newer authors, however, are careful to distinguish between management and leadership. In their review of the literature, Gregoire and Arendt noted that managers seek order and control, whereas leaders thrive on chaos and seek ways to attain goals while coping with change.[23] This important distinction is important for the advanced practice dietitian, who may lead an organization or group laterally rather than from a position of control. Many great leaders, including Mohandas Ghandi and Martin Luther King, Jr., did not occupy a formal leadership or management position. Likewise, advanced practice dietitians may not lead movements resulting in great social change, but may still learn lateral leadership techniques that advance themselves, their practices, or the dietetics profession as a whole.

When Gregoire and Arendt reviewed the leadership literature from the dietetics perspective, they concluded that the dietetics profession needs leaders.[23] They also pointed out that more information on leadership in dietetics is needed, because most of the currently available data are descriptive. For example, Schiller et al. surveyed more than 1100 clinical nutrition managers who attended invitational leadership workshops and concluded that a cadre of self-actualized leaders existed, but that many dietitians avoided leadership, seeking security rather than satisfaction.[24] In a follow-up study of 150 clinical managers, Arensberg et al. found that managers rated themselves higher than did their subordinates on a validated leadership behavior questionnaire.[25] Results showed that managers were respectful, but scored lower on communication.

Letos et al. surveyed graduates of a program to train dietetics practitioners in maternal and child nutrition.[26] This program emphasized leadership as evidenced by participation in nutrition organizations and publications in the scientific literature. The results of this study suggested that leadership activities can be learned and taught at the post-professional level. In fact, 93% of the graduates of this program participated in leadership activities following program completion. Leadership activities listed by the study participants included building collaborative relationships, developing programs, advocacy, and participation in local nutrition organizations.

In discussing their results, Arensberg et al. suggest that publications and presentations correlated with positive leadership styles.[25] Other researchers have proposed that career advancement, salary, or numbers of employees might be used as objective measures of leadership. Still others focus on more intangible dimensions of leadership, such as one's sphere of influence or emotional maturity. Clearly, the dimensions of leadership in advanced practice dietetics require further discussion and definition before widespread agreement is achieved. However, an example that leaders might identify with is found in **Exhibit 6–4.**

EXHIBIT 6–4

Leadership in Clinic Participation

Early in my career, I encountered a couple of patients with celiac disease. The diet was complicated and the patients were interesting, but the disease was thought to be rare. Years later, I came across an article that addressed the fact that celiac disease was under diagnosed and much more common than originally thought. It contained some figures suggesting that we would have about one case a week diagnosed in the smallish city where I lived. It also mentioned a lab test that looked promising. Of course the only really effective treatment is diet, so I learned all that I could about the diet and available food products. Then I set up meetings with two of the busiest gastroenterologists in our area. I shared what I had read and asked if they were seeing more patients with symptoms similar to those described in the article. One said he had no

continues

EXHIBIT 6–4 *continued*

interest in these patients, and the other said he just told his patients not to eat gluten. I talked with the second physician for a while, and I could tell that he was becoming interested in what I had to say. I offered to see patients for him in my office. Things went well with the first two or three patients. I developed a simple system to measure and record their increased knowledge of what foods to eat and avoid, their satisfaction with nutritional management, and their improved symptoms. Soon, I was being consulted often enough that I began my own clinic days in the physician's office. Now, I'm there two days a week and see patients for another physician as well. I'm lucky not only to have come across that article, but to have the leadership skills to move my practice forward.

Leadership: A Summary

The formal study of leadership may be new to dietitians, but advanced practice dietitians exhibit leadership skills. These skills are used to create advanced practice roles and to bring others into these roles.

AWARENESS

"Let us not look back in anger or forward in fear, but around in awareness."
—James Thurber[27]

Awareness may be defined as having or showing realization, perception, or knowledge.[3] The dietitians in our study possessed extensive knowledge of self, the work setting, and the greater environment. They exhibited a keen awareness of political and regulatory influences within their environment. In addition, they understood how they influenced both the environment and the boundaries of that environment. These dietitians were aware of not only organizational issues, but also their role within the organization. They challenged administrative structures or created their own structures as needed; during this process, they exhibited finely developed political skills, which they used to obtain cooperation and support for their initiatives. One advised other dietitians to "evaluate the system and its effectiveness and enter into the system as you need to." Awareness was also expressed in the following way: "Sometimes you can't change things because you don't have control over certain things, but at least you share the information and work with your group toward that end." In keeping with these perceptions, the following discussion of awareness is divided into three areas: self-awareness, organizational awareness, and situational awareness.

Self-Awareness

Self-awareness is essential to advanced practice. Golman includes awareness as one of the self-management skills needed for emotional intelligence.[28] He characterizes self-aware individuals as being knowledgeable of their weaknesses and able to plan around them. Borrell-Carrio and Epstein take self-awareness a step farther, applying the concept to a strategy for reducing errors in diagnostic judgment.[29] Both of these models apply to dietitians as they move into more responsible roles, including nutrition diagnosis.

Self-aware individuals know what triggers their behavior and are able to predict how they will react in specific situations. They are aware of their value systems and often select situations that are compatible with their values. Self-awareness is a key to productivity because it enables people to select activities, jobs, or careers that are compatible with their personalities.

Organizational Awareness

The advanced practice dietitian's awareness does not stop with self, but extends to the surrounding organization as well. Organizational awareness has been defined as knowing the organization's mission and functions; understanding how its social, political, and technological systems work; and operating effectively within those systems. Further, organizational awareness includes the programs, policies, procedures, rules, and regulations of the organization.[30] See Exhibit 6–5.

Organizational awareness is essential if advanced practice dietitians hope to establish and expand their roles. The advanced practice dietitian is familiar with the term "corporate culture," which describes an approach to work held in common by successful workers within the organization. Corporate culture may extend to issues such as dress, punctuality, speech patterns, structure of meetings, adherence to work schedules, and work standards. In addition, more subtle differences are centered on corporate leadership and power. Geographic influences are also important. For example, healthcare institutions in the Northeast and some parts of the South tend to be more conservative, employing a formal hierarchical approach. By contrast, in the Midwest, a more relaxed, egalitarian atmosphere prevails. In other areas, a more liberal and informal professional environment exists.

One advanced practice dietitian contrasted two previous employers by stating that one was concerned about how things "looked" whereas the other was concerned with how things "were." Another noted the following differences in organizations:

> There are differences in organizational structure, and who holds power. In one hospital, surgeons may control most of the resources, while in another, the power of the medical staff is palpable. In some organizations, accountants or other managers exercise great authority, while in others nursing or other groups of clinicians have a deep voice.

Most advanced practice dietitians are not only aware of internal factors such as the number of staff available, but are also aware of how these factors are controlled. Such dietitians know the organization's policies and procedures but—more importantly—understand how those policies and procedures are derived and changed. These professionals anticipate recurring events, such as employee evaluations and inspections, and consider their impact on organizational resources and decision making. For example, the advanced practice dietitian knows when the fiscal year ends, when budget negotiations are conducted, and what the organizational focus is—that is, the reigning influence on decision making, whether quality, marketing, patient satisfaction, reducing costs, or increasing revenue.

The advanced practice dietitian anticipates the effects of state and federal policies, political events, and news stories, and is knowledgeable about how these events will influence decisions. He or she is also aware of the revenue streams, case mix, and other economic drivers of practice that accompany the referral base. Such a professional is acutely aware of the referral base for the organization, whether it is a hospital, long-term care facility, clinic, or private practice. The advanced practice dietitian knows which physicians want nutrition input and which physicians do not, and why. More importantly, the advanced practice dietitian is able to operate effectively within these constraints, using them as bases on which to develop initiatives and improve practice outcomes.

Situational Awareness

Situational awareness has been simply described as knowing what is going on around you or as having an awareness of environmental cues.[31] This type of awareness is used to deal with a broad array and volume of changing data. It involves the correct integration and interpretation of data related to a goal and task. Situational awareness is used by pilots, for example, to describe the large number of variables known to affect their cognitive performance. It is also applied in engineering, security, and counterterrorism. In health care, situational awareness is a key tool for improving quality and reducing errors.

Situational awareness is used wherever quick and complex thinking is needed. In dietetics, this kind of awareness may relate to the process of filtering information from patients, families, caregivers, the scientific literature, and guidelines so as to develop an appropriate and meaningful solution or plan for the case at hand. In this sort of scenario, analysis of complex factors is needed even as the dietitian focuses on what is important or what will make a difference. In the short term, this kind of awareness may be evident within a single conversation with another health professional on rounds. Alternatively, it may involve a greater set of dynamic situations within a group or organization.

Awareness: A Summary

The advanced practice dietitian's awareness includes knowledge of self, the organization, and the situation. The advanced practice dietitian applies this knowledge effectively in complex and changing situations. The result of such awareness is improved accuracy, productivity, and effectiveness.

EXHIBIT 6–5

Awareness of Political and Policy Influences

And probably half of who I am today is just because I've been involved in the dietetic association. I think it adds to my comfort to myself who I am. So at any given time, I can pick up the phone and call and contact somebody to make a difference. So I don't know whether you remember back when the FDA came out and made their statement about infant formulas? I'm the one that, because I worked with the pediatric nutrition practice group, knew to make the call to ADA and to let them know that ADA needed to be involved. They needed to be a speaker on this topic. It's not that we don't have strong leadership. It's just that they didn't necessarily have that connection. They weren't aware of the importance of the FDA statement and how we needed to be involved. I had worked with a couple of policy issues at the state level and knew the influence we could have if we were able to respond. And we did. We made a difference. If I hadn't known how ADA worked, it would have been much more difficult to have an impact.

SUMMARY

The advanced practice dietitian does not work in isolation, but rather applies himself or herself within the context of a larger environment. Such a dietitian is influenced by this environment and, in turn, uses the elements of the context sub-theme to interact with the professional environment. Using skills geared toward collaboration, networking, consultation, leadership, and awareness, the advanced practice dietitian in MNT influences both patients (either alone or in groups) and the environment of practice.

KEY POINTS

- Advanced practice dietitians use the context sub-themes to maximize their effectiveness as part of the healthcare team.
- They use interdisciplinary collaboration and participate fully in shared decision making to improve effectiveness.
- They engage in networking with dietitians and other health professionals to obtain information and solve problems.
- Advanced practice dietitians have adopted the consultation and referral mechanism to increase the value of their services.
- They use leadership to initiate and manage change at different levels.
- Advanced practice dietitians use awareness of self, organizations, and situations to maximize outcomes.

SUGGESTED READING

Collaboration

Baker DP, Gustafson S, Beaubien J, Salas E, Barach P. *Medical teamwork and patient safety: The evidence-based relation.* AHRQ Publication No. 05-0053. Rockville, MD: Agency for Healthcare Research and Quality, April 005. Available at http://www.ahrq.gov/qual/medteam/.

This extensive resource is available for free online from the Agency for Healthcare Research and Quality.

Conflict Resolution Network. Available at http://www.crnhq.org/. Accessed February 13, 2007.

This site contains a summary of 12 skills for conflict resolution that may help in developing your own and other people's behavior.

Johnson R, Eaton J. *Influencing people.* London: Dorling Kindersly, 2002.

This brief text quickly summarizes how to get our message across to others.

Mindell P. *How to say it for women*. New York: Prentice Hall, 2001.

This text will help you understand how to be more effective in communicating your recommendations.

Networking

Career Journal.com. Available at http://www.careerjournal.com/jobhunting/networking/20050215-bradford.html. Accessed March 13, 2007.

This site is sponsored by the *Wall Street Journal* and offers a series of easy-to-read articles about networking. It's geared toward finding a job, but the techniques discussed here also apply to other situations.

Ferrazzi K, Raz T. *Never eat alone: And other secrets to success, one relationship at a time*. New York: Random House, 2005.

A popular, easy-to-read book about building business relationships.

Leadership

Bushe G. Appreciative leadership. *Journal of the American Dietetic Association* 2005;105(5): 699–700.

Leadership applied to dietetics by one of the speakers at ADA's Leadership Institute.

Bushe GR. *Clear leadership*. Palo Alto, CA: Davies-Black, 2001.

A brief and practical approach to leadership.

Collins JC. *Good to great*. New York: HarperCollins, 2001.

A popular book on leadership among healthcare executives.

Goleman D. What makes a leader? *Harvard Business Review* 1998;76:93–102.

A readable academic resource.

Heifetz RA. *Leadership without easy answers*. Cambridge, MA: Belknap Press of Harvard University Press, 1994.

This text, which comes from the Harvard Leadership Institute, is an academic but readable text that integrates leadership theory and practice.

Smith D, Bell GD, Kilgo J. *The Carolina way*. New York: Penguin Books, 2004.

For sports fans, this is an interesting approach to management and leadership from Dean Smith, the successful University of North Carolina basketball coach.

Awareness

BestFit.com. Available at http://www.bestfittype.com/.

Information on personality types, including a section on "what it is like to be me." Links to books for purchase that provide more detail and explain interactions between the different personality types related to job and career issues.

Buckingham M, Clifton DO. *Discover your strengths*. New York: Free Press, 2001.

This book helps people to become aware of their strengths. It comes with a unique number that allows access to an online "strength finder" instrument.

Keirsey D. *Please understand me II*. Del Mar: Prometheus Nemesis, 1998.

This book combines a simplified test instrument based on the Myers–Briggs Type Inventory with more detail about the 16 personality types.

Myers–Briggs Foundation. Available at http://www.myersbriggs.org/my-mbti-personality-type/mbti-basics/the-16-mbti-types.asp.

This website contains an overview of the 16 personality types identified by Katherine Meyers and Isabel Briggs as well as resources for how to use personality types to better communicate.

EXPERIENCES TO TRY

Collaboration

1. Look up the Nursing Scope of Practice, Pharmacy Scope of Practice, Physician Assistant Scope of Practice, and Physical Therapy Scope of Practice for your state. These documents will be posted on the websites of the agency in your state that regulates healthcare practice. Compare these documents with the Scope of Practice for Dietitians in your state. What are your observations?

2. Obtain a copy of the American College of Clinical Pharmacy's "Position Statement: Collaborative Drug Therapy Management by Pharmacists—2003" (available at http://www.accp.com/position.php#positionstatements; accessed February 14, 2007). After reading it, can you envision such a model in dietetics? In your own practice? How does this document compare with the ADA's position on pharmacotherapy and nutrition?

3. At the end of each day, list the people with whom you interact. Take a few minutes to reflect on how these interactions could have been more positive. What techniques can you use to achieve more positive results?

4. Make a list of three or four groups to which you belong. List the contributions you have made to each group within the last 12 months (other than attending the meetings). Plan how you can improve your contributions in the future. Is there an empty niche you can fill? Do you have skills that the group needs, but that you are not providing? Are you participating to your full potential?

Networking

1. Plan to introduce yourself at a meeting or networking event. Prepare an "elevator speech"—that is, practice what you would like others to know

about you in 30 seconds or less. Describe what an advanced practice dietitian does; describe your particular skill set.

2. Join a new group. See how many people you can meet. Make it a point to meeting new people at each gathering. Listen to their "elevator speeches." Can you identify the formal and informal leaders of the group? Can you identify an opportunity to participate? What role could you play? Afterward, try to think of how you might collaborate in the future with the new people you meet.

Leadership

1. Do you have a personal mission, vision, and values statement? If so, revisit it and see if the statement is still meaningful. If not, try writing one. Try the mission statement tool at http://www.franklincovey.com/fc/library_and_resources/mission_statement_builder.

2. Think of a change that is needed in your professional or work life. Begin to think of how you might use leadership skills to make this change happen. Would you get a group together, present information on the issue, and obtain input from the group? How would you involve people in your process? Who would be needed to support or lead the change? What information would you need to make changes? Start small, develop your leadership skills, and then move on to larger projects.

Awareness

1. Make a calendar for recurring events, such as inspections, evaluations, and events that stress your boss or your organization. Can you see how to plan major projects or time requests around that timeline?

2. Locate your department's or organization's mission statement. Compare it to your own mission statement. Are there differences? Make a list of the major issues facing your organization. Ask your boss for input on this task. Ask key people with whom you interact for their input into the list. Are the issues the same for all groups?

3. Develop a perspective on the regulations governing your practice. Review your state licensure laws and scope of practice for dietitians, the ADA Scope of Practice documents, and the Standards for Professional Performance for your particular specialty. What would you change? Who would you approach about a change? How would you convince others to support the change you propose?

4. If you haven't done so already, take the Myers–Briggs Type Indicator. Have the test scored and review the results. Consider whether the personality identified by this instrument feels authentic for you. Read about your personality type, and think about how it affects you within your professional environment.

5. Learn what the people around you read, and review those publications or websites. Become familiar with the issues that are important to people around you.

REFERENCES

1. Saarinen E. Quote. *Time*. Available at http://www.researchover.com/quotes/keywords/context/. Accessed April 17, 2007.
2. Creativity quotes. Available at http://www.mycoted.com/Creativity_Quotes. Accessed March 13, 2007.
3. Merriam-Webster Online. Available at www.m-w.com/. Accessed July 5, 2006.
4. *Health professions education: A bridge to quality.* Washington, DC: Institute of Medicine, 2003.
5. Nugent KE, Lambert VA. The advanced practice nurse in collaborative practice. *Nursing Connections* 1996;9(1):5–16.
6. Lindeke LL, Block DE. Maintaining professional integrity in the midst of interdisciplinary collaboration. *Nursing Outlook* 1998;46(5):213–218.
7. Skipper A, Lewis NM. Using initiative to achieve autonomy: A model for advanced medical nutrition therapy practice. *Journal of the American Dietetic Association* 2006;106(8):1219–1225.
8. Institute of Medicine. Crossing the quality chasm: A new health system for the 21st century. Washington, DC: Institute of Medicine, 2001.
9. *2006 comprehensive accreditation manual for hospitals: The official handbook.* Oakbrook, IL: Joint Commission, 2006.
10. Leape LL, Cullen DJ, Clapp MD, et al. Pharmacist participation on physician rounds and adverse drug events in the intensive care unit. *Journal of the American Medical Association* 1999;282(3):267–270.
11. Gattis WA, Hasselblad V, Whellan DJ, O'Connor C. Reduction in heart failure events by the addition of a clinical pharmacist to the heart failure management team: Results of the Pharmacist in Heart Failure Assessment Recommendation and Monitoring (PHARM) study. *Archives of Internal Medicine* 1999;159(16):1939–1945.
12. Isetts BJ, Brown LM, Schondelmeyer SW, Lenarz LA. Quality assessment of a collaborative approach for decreasing drug-related morbidity and achieving therapeutic goals. *Archives of Internal Medicine* 2003;163(15):1813–1820.
13. Dutton RP, Cooper C, Jones A, Leone S, Kramer ME, Scalea TM. Daily multidisciplinary rounds shorten length of stay for trauma patients. *Journal of Trauma* 2003;55(5):913–919.
14. Sommers LS, Marton KI, Barbaccia JD, Randolph J. Physician, nurse, and social worker collaboration in primary care for chronically ill seniors. *Archives of Internal Medicine* 2000;160(12):1825–1833.

15. Mensing C, Boucher J, Cypress M, et al. National standards for diabetes self-management education. *Diabetes Care* 2000;23(5):682–689.
16. Brainy quote. Available at http://www.brainyquote.com/. Accessed March 13, 2007.
17. West E, Barron, DN, Dowsett J, Bewton JN. Hierarchies and cliques in the social networks of health care professionals: Implications for the design of dissemination strategies. *Social Science and Medicine* 1999;48(5):633–646.
18. Hill R, Dunbar R. Social network size in humans. *Human Nature* 2002;14(1):53–72.
19. Bradley RT, Young WY, Ebbs P, Martin J. Characteristics of advanced-level dietetics practice: A model and empirical results. *Journal of the American Dietetic Association* 1993;93:196–202.
20. Skipper A, Young M, Rotman N, Nagl H. Physicians' implementation of dietitians' recommendations: A study of the effectiveness of dietitians. *Journal of the American Dietetic Association* 1994;94(1):45–49.
21. Heifetz RA. *Leadership without easy answers.* Cambridge, MA: Belknap Press of Harvard University Press, 1994.
22. Smith Edge M. All ADA members are leaders. *Journal of the American Dietetic Association* 2003;103(11):1452.
23. Gregoire MB, Arendt SW. Leadership: Reflections over the past 100 years. *Journal of the American Dietetic Association* 2004;104(3):395–403.
24. Schiller MR, Foltz MB, Campbell SM. Dietitians' self-perceptions: Implications for leadership. *Journal of the American Dietetic Association* 1993;93(8):868–874.
25. Arensberg MBF, Schiller MR, Vivian VM, Strasser S. Transformational leadership of clinical nutrition managers. *Journal of the American Dietetic Association* 1996;96(1): 39–45.
26. Letos SN, Trahms CM, Lucas B, Powell JA. Maternal and child health nutrition training builds leadership skills. *Journal of the American Dietetic Association* 2001;101(5): 567–571.
27. Wisdom quotes. Available at http://www.wisdomquotes.com/002629.html. Accessed April 17, 2007.
28. Goleman D. What makes a leader? *Harvard Business Review* 1998;76(6):93–102.
29. Borrell-Carrio F, Epstein RM. Preventing errors in clinical practice: A call for self awareness. *Annals of Family Medicine* 2004;2(4):310–316.
30. Transportation Security Administration. Awareness. Available at http://www.tsa.gov/join/benefits/editorial_1499.shtm. Accessed September 22, 2006.
31. Endsley MR. Theoretical underpinnings of situation awareness: A critical review. In Endsley MR, Garland DJ (eds.). *Situation awareness analysis and measurement.* Mahwah, NJ: Lawrence Erlbaum Associates, 2000.

Advanced Practice Expertise

"I offer my expertise and experience for hire in order to help a group of people reach the summit." —Anatoli Boukreev[1]

Many of the skills described in the previous chapters are transferable across professions. For example, leadership is taught in business and agriculture schools. Awareness is used in the transportation and safety industries as well as in the military. Certainly collaboration and creativity are widely used to solve problems and develop products in the electronics and technology industries. These and other skills in the context and attitude sub-themes of the advanced MNT model serve as a sort of "envelope" that surrounds the unique core of MNT expertise. In this chapter, we address the sub-theme that describes the core skills that are unique to the expertise of the advanced practice dietitian. As mentioned previously, it is the expert performance of advanced practice MNT skills that distinguishes the advanced practice dietitian from other dietitians and from other health professionals.

At first glance, dietitians may see similarities between the advanced medical nutrition skills and the tasks that are performed at the basic or specialty level of practice. Careful examination reveals that these skills are not included in the basic educational competencies required for dietetic registration. Although some of these topics may be given cursory treatment in baccalaureate programs, in internships, or in seminars offered as continuing education, it is unlikely that a baccalaureate degree program in dietetics, a dietetic internship, or a continuing education offering will be of sufficient depth and duration to provide the level of understanding that constitutes true expertise. To wit, advanced MNT expertise is both broader and deeper than basic level knowledge, and it is accompanied by extensive graduate-level education and years of practice experience.

The Centers for Medicare and Medicaid Services has defined *medical nutrition therapy* as "nutrition diagnostic, therapy, and counseling services for the purpose of disease management which are furnished by a registered dietitian or nutrition professional."[2] The ADA adds that MNT is specific to the Nutrition Care Process in clinical* settings. It further states that MNT involves in-depth, individualized nutrition assessment and a duration and frequency of care using the Nutrition Care Process to manage disease.[3]

"Medical nutrition therapy" is a relatively new term. It appeared in the early 1990s as dietitians began to actively pursue reimbursement for their services. MNT

---

*A clinical setting is any location in which direct patient or client care is provided. It includes, but is not limited to, acute care hospitals, outpatient clinics, congregate feeding sites, physicians' offices, long-term care, WIC and other public health clinics, assisted living, rehabilitation facilities, behavioral health facilities, and drug and food stores.

is a unique function whose conduct is the sole province of the dietetics profession; no other profession has the depth of education or experience required to provide this kind of therapy. MNT does not refer to normal nutrition or healthy eating, which is part of lifestyle advice provided to the general public by dietitians, other health professionals, and unlicensed practitioners. Instead, MNT is a specific intervention designed to improve the outcome for a specific nutrition diagnosis.

Advanced practice dietitians independently provide MNT without supervision by another dietitian or a member of another profession such as a nurse or physician. In short, they deliver MNT at a level of expertise, autonomy, and responsibility consistent with the level of expertise exhibited by an experienced practitioner in any profession.

The distinction between advanced practice dietitians and entry-level dietitians was described by one dietitian in the following way:

> [Entry-level dietitians are] coming out of school with textbook learning, and they are memorizing scales, formulas, calculations, and biochemistry—but not the multifaceted level of care that people with chronic disease need. The problem-solving things that are necessary could be taught and would be very beneficial [but] I don't think [they are] currently being taught in any of the dietetics programs.

Another advanced practice dietitian stated, "Basic level dietitians practice the 'right way' to do things. They search out a single best approach. When they are presented with a situation that does not fit into their notion of what's right, they will search for a rule to help them out." In the words of one advanced practitioner, "Basic level practitioners look for rules so that they won't make a mistake. Advanced practitioners have the knowledge and skill to make those rules. Then they have the courage to change them as they learn more." Clearly, advanced practice dietitians understand the concepts supporting practice and know that the right way to do things varies based on the needs of the particular situation and the needs of the particular patient.

Based on interviews with advanced practitioners and the results of at least one survey, there appear to be specific areas of expertise for the advanced practice dietitian that can be taught in the classroom and in the patient or client setting,[4,5] namely, nutrition pharmacology, nutrition pathophysiology, advanced MNT, nutrition co-morbidities, and nutrition outcomes research. This chapter briefly discusses each of these sub-themes, clarifying how advanced practitioners in these areas differ from the basic and specialty levels of practice, providing examples of MNT expertise as described by advanced practice dietitians, and proposing courses or topics that might be developed to enhance the expertise of the advanced practice dietitian practicing in MNT.

NUTRITION PHARMACOLOGY

"Let your food be medicine and your medicine be food." —Hippocrates[6]

The word "pharmacology" is derived from two Greek words: *pharmakos,* meaning "drug," and *logos,* meaning "science."[7] *Pharmacology* has been defined as the science of drugs, including their origin, composition, pharmacokinetics, therapeutic use, and toxicology.[8] *Nutrition* has been defined as the relationship between diet and health.[7] With these definitions of nutrition and pharmacology in mind, we can explore the definition of nutrition pharmacology.

The term *nutrition pharmacology* is used differently by different users. Drug companies use this term to describe the unique nutritional profile of a product. Nutritionists use it to describe the practice of giving large amounts of nutrients to achieve a therapeutic effect. Medical school curricula include courses or lectures on nutrition pharmacology. A review of syllabi for these courses, however, reveals that they discuss drugs that affect gastrointestinal function or lipid profiles; few, if any, cover even the most basic nutrition information.

The advanced practice dietitians interviewed in our study referred to nutrition pharmacology as the manipulation of foods, nutrients, and nutrition-related drugs by a registered dietitian in collaboration with other health providers. A proposed definition of nutrition pharmacology relative to advanced practice in dietetics is "a discipline in which the goal is to balance nutrient intake and drug dose so as to optimize the therapeutic effects of both nutrients and drugs and thereby improve the health of the patient."

In basic level practice, dietitians memorize lists of drug–nutrient interactions and restrict the intake of the offending nutrients in the diet. For example, basic level dietitians know that green leafy vegetables are a source of vitamin K, so they tell patients who are receiving anticoagulation therapy to avoid them. They do not typically appreciate the differences between the types of anticoagulants or their mechanisms of action, however. Lacking this knowledge, basic level dietitians may unnecessarily instruct patients to refrain from eating some favorite foods. In contrast, the advanced practice dietitian begins by determining whether the anticoagulant is one that requires vitamin K restriction. Such a dietitian understands the differences in the mechanisms of action of the various anticoagulants and recognizes the indications, contraindications, side effects, and duration of action for each medication. The advanced practice dietitian can discuss the vitamin K interactions with each anticoagulant with the pharmacist, physician, and nurse; he or she can also explain these drug–nutrient interactions to the patient. Finally, the advanced practice dietitian effectively counsels the patient according to his or her unique food preferences and level of understanding about the foods to eat or avoid while taking anticoagulants.

Nutrition pharmacology is a growing area of importance in MNT. The number of drugs introduced each year and the number of prescriptions written each year for patients have steadily increased.[9] Not surprisingly, given these trends, the advanced practice dietitian often encounters patients who are taking complex drug regimens. Many of the drugs in these regimens can interact with a variety of food and nutrients. For example, some may increase (or decrease) metabolic rate, others may improve (or impede) appetite, and still others may enhance (or inhibit) nutrient absorption.[10–12] Some drugs contain substantial amounts of nutrients, such as potassium, sodium, or lipids.

In the intensive care unit, dietitians often calculate the fluids and other nutrients provided in drugs and adapt the composition and timing of enteral and parenteral feedings accordingly. Some dietitians who work with critically ill patients have developed expert knowledge of the effects of nutrient-wasting drugs, hypoglycemic agents, and drugs that cause hyperglycemia. Advanced practice dietitians may manipulate nutrient intake in concert with drugs that alter gastrointestinal motility, nutrient absorption, or nutrient metabolism. In many hospitals, advanced practice dietitians order both parenteral nutrition and other drugs that are part of the parenteral admixture.[13,14]

Dietitians who work with patients who have chronic, debilitating diseases may recommend and implement appetite stimulants. In institutional settings, these professionals may work closely with nurses and pharmacists to coordinate the timing of medications and meals. In ambulatory settings or clinics, dietitians may review medication profiles and teach patients how to schedule meals and medications.

In settings where pharmacists are not always available, dietitians have assumed responsibility for managing nutrient-related drugs in addition to food and nutrient intake. In some settings, dietitians have obtained clinical privileges allowing them to adjust drugs, thereby streamlining care and improving patient convenience.[15] For example, in dialysis centers, dietitians often manage phosphate binders, iron therapy, and vitamin D supplementation by adjusting these medications' doses based on laboratory data and nutrient intake. In diabetes clinics, dietitians typically identify and correct problems caused by an imbalance between food intake and hypoglycemic agents.[16,17] Indeed, as part of their credentialing examination, Board Certified–Advanced Diabetes Managers are tested on their ability to select, initiate, and adjust pharmacotherapy.[18]

Advanced practice dietitians in our study mentioned manipulating food and nutrients in response to drug therapy more often than any other intervention. One dietitian working in a dialysis center "developed Epogen [Amgen; epoetin alfa] protocols and did Calcijex [Abbott Laboratories; calcitriol] and Zemplar [Abbott Laboratories; paracalcitol] protocols and IV irons and phosphate binders." Another dietitian stated that advanced practice dietitians "make medication recommendations that are supported by the treating physician." In another facility, dietitians wrote orders for insulin, histamine-receptor antagonists, and other parenteral drugs that were administered as additives to parenteral nutrition.

The dietitians in the study maintained a high level of expertise related to the drugs used, easily discussing the mechanism of action and relative advantages and disadvantages of different types of insulin, the properties of various antiemetics, and the relative value of therapeutic doses of nutrients in specific diseases or conditions. One dietitian attended annual pharmacology updates to keep abreast of new drugs applicable to her patient population. Others regularly attended in-service educational programs or read drug newsletters to maintain awareness of available drugs and their nutritional implications.

Given their high level of involvement in coping with potential drug–nutrient interactions and the frequency with which this responsibility was mentioned, advanced practice dietitians may consider obtaining additional education and training in the pharmacologic effects and interactions of food and nutrients. In a survey of experienced dietitians, respondents expressed a high level of interest in nutrition pharmacology coursework. Thus it appears that there is a real need for dietitians to study pharmacology as part of an advanced practice curriculum. It is unknown how many graduate programs currently offer the opportunity for students to take courses in pharmacology. **Table 7–1** shows a proposed outline for a course in nutrition pharmacology. **Exhibit 7–1** provides an example of how nutrition pharmacology is applied in the clinical setting.

Clearly, advanced practice dietitians possess the depth and breadth of knowledge required to manipulate food, nutrients, and drugs and thereby improve patients' health. These skills, which collectively constitute nutrition pharmacology, were the most frequently mentioned of a wide range of skills exhibited by advanced practice dietitians. It appears that there is an ample body of knowledge and interest to support a graduate-level course in nutrition pharmacology.

Table 7–1 A Proposed Outline for a Graduate-Level Nutrition Pharmacology Course

Basic Pharmaceutical Principles
   Drug Delivery and Administration (Dosage Forms)
Overview of Pharmacokinetics
   Drug Absorption, Distribution, Metabolism, and Excretion
Overview of Pharmacodynamics
   Drug Actions
Biopharmaceutics of Orally Ingested Products
   Relationships Between Food and Drug Ingestion
Laws Governing Drug Development, Marketing, and Prescribing
Nutritional Implications of Drugs
   Neurological and Central Nervous System Drugs
   Anti-inflammatory Drugs
   Renal and Cardiovascular Drugs
   Gastrointestinal Drugs
   Antimicrobials
   Antineoplastic Drugs
   Immunomodulators
   Drugs Affecting Blood and Blood-Forming Organs
   Hormones and Hormone Antagonists
   Parenteral Nutrition
Nutritional Implications of Nonprescription Drugs and Supplements
   Caffeine
   Alcohol
Nutrients Used as Drugs
   Vitamins and Minerals
   Amino Acids
Prebiotics and Probiotics
Herbs and Botanicals

NUTRITION PATHOPHYSIOLOGY

"Whatsoever was the father of disease, an ill diet was the mother." —*Unknown*[19]

Pathophysiology is defined as the study (Greek: *logos*) or science of suffering (Greek: *pathos*).[20] Thus *nutrition pathophysiology* may be defined as the study of suffering related to nutrition. Nutrition pathophysiology should provide the link between

EXHIBIT 7–1

Identifying Inadequate Glycemic Control Using a Food and Nutrition History

I sometimes find problems with drugs, especially insulin. For instance, an elderly man was referred to me because his blood sugars were high. The doctor was sure he wasn't compliant with the diet. When they sent the patient to me, the first thing I noticed was how thin he was. I said to him, "Okay, I want you to give me a feel for what you're eating in a day." He went through what he ate. He was eating like a bird, yet his blood sugars were in the 300s. If I hadn't known all the things I learned as an advanced practitioner, I would have done diet teaching—but I knew that's not what his problem was. The problem was that the patient needed to be on insulin. His pills (oral hypoglycemic agents) weren't doing the job for him, and he was starving himself trying to be compliant with the doctor's edict to get his blood sugar down.

Fortunately, I knew the nurse over in the diabetic clinic, and had heard her say she had a cancellation that afternoon. I picked up the phone and said, "I've got a patient here who I'm sure needs insulin. Can you get him into your clinic this afternoon?" Sure enough, they started him on insulin. When he came back in a month, he had gained 15 pounds. He felt much better.

normal nutrition and the nutrition abnormalities causing or resulting from disease. It is the process by which nutrition-related disease occurs. Nutrition pathophysiology includes deficiencies or excesses in food and nutrient intake as well as abnormalities in nutrient absorption, metabolism, and excretion. This discipline should be considered a specialized form of pathology that focuses on specific organs' and tissues' responses to inadequate or excess food and nutrient intake. As such, it includes the genetic, molecular, biochemical, microbiological, immunologic, and morphologic bases for altered absorption, metabolism, and excretion.

Nutrition scientists have focused almost exclusively on identifying nutrient requirements and describing normal nutrient metabolism. Despite this emphasis, it is well known that numerous diseases—including hypertension, obesity, cardiovascular disease, and diabetes—are closely related to abnormalities of nutrient intake. More recently, nutrition epidemiologists have attempted to elucidate the food and nutrient intake factors associated with these diseases. The work of these two groups (i.e., nutrition scientists and epidemiologists) has made obvious the void of information about how nutritional disease develops at the cellular level and within an individual patient. Clearly, an understanding of nutrition pathophysiology is needed to effectively identify and treat nutritional diseases. A model that categorizes nutrition pathologic processes into food and nutrient intake, absorption, metabolism, and excretion can, therefore, be used to examine available knowledge.

Intake

Optimal nutrition occurs when the amount of food and nutrients consumed equals the amount required for each individual, regardless of his or her age and state of wellness or disease. Nevertheless, differences in requirements and intake are prevalent at a number of levels. For example, the Food and Agriculture Organization of the United Nations has identified one of its goals as decreasing the number of undernourished people worldwide from 800 million to 400 million.[21] In the United States, food insecurity is a well-recognized problem,[22] and malnutrition is known to occur at a relatively high rate in children, the elderly, and persons with chronic disease.[23,24] In U.S. healthcare institutions, the incidence of malnutrition is typically greater than 30%.[25]

At the other end of the spectrum, the abundance of cheap food in the United States and other developed countries has given rise to a growing problem of obesity and related diseases such as diabetes and cancer. The prevalence of obesity in developed countries may approach 45%.

Thus a large percentage of the U.S. population experiences either inadequate or excess food and nutrient intake. Advanced practice dietitians can provide sophisticated interventions to these individuals or populations so as to reduce the gap between actual and ideal intake.

Absorption

The study of nutrient absorption has expanded in the last decade, in part owing to the identification of new markers of gastrointestinal function. As a result of the discovery of these improved biomarkers of nutrient absorption, increasing numbers of patients have been diagnosed with malabsorptive diseases such as celiac disease.

Advanced practice dietitians will need to stay current with new biomarkers for nutrient absorption and the results of research generated using these tests if they are to develop effective interventions for treating malabsorption.

Metabolism

The study of nutrient metabolism is evolving into one of metabolomics. That is, using genetic testing, the nutrient metabolism of an individual can be discerned and used to design individualized nutrient interventions.[26] For example, studies have identified genetic differences in metabolism of HDL cholesterol and adiposity.[27,28] This work represents merely the beginning; hundreds of studies will undoubtedly be launched that will define an entire new field with important implications for dietitians. Advanced practice dietitians will find it necessary to keep up with these studies and to improve and individualize nutrition interventions based on their findings.

Excretion

Nutrient excretion varies depending on nutrient intake, nutrient absorption, and the health of the organs involved in nutrient metabolism. For example, protein is conserved and adaptive mechanisms attempt to preserve muscle during periods of restricted protein intake, whereas protein excretion is impaired in renal disease and nitrogen is retained in liver disease. These factors have important ramifications for MNT and the amount and type of nutrient intake prescribed. The intake–absorption–metabolism–excretion model can be used to increase understanding of both macronutrients and micronutrients: Understanding of these four factors relative to individual nutrients enables the advanced practice dietitian to adapt therapy to the least complex and most effective form.

The intake–absorption–metabolism–excretion model may be applied to nutrient aberrations, as seen in **Table 7–2**. The same model might also be used along with material from the current literature to develop a graduate-level course in nutrition pathophysiology. A proposed outline for such a course appears in **Table 7–3**. Although this list of topics is based on the most common causes of disease and illness in the United States, other diseases might be added as necessary or desired. It is unknown whether courses in nutrient pathophysiology are widely available, but graduate-level courses most likely focus on normal nutrient metabolism rather than on nutrient metabolism in disease. Knowledge of normal nutrient metabolism is a prerequisite for nutrition pathophysiology, but knowledge of normal

Table 7–2 Application of the Intake–Absorption–Metabolism–Excretion Model to Phosphorus in Health and Renal Disease

Normal Nutrition	Nutrition Pathophysiology
Intake	**Intake**
The DRI for phosphorus with supporting research	Trends in phosphorus consumption with packaged foods and the effect of increased phosphorus intake on renal stone formation and chronic renal failure
Food sources of phosphorus	
Absorption	**Absorption**
Percentage of phosphorus absorbed from food	Absorptive changes with excess or inadequate intake or with renal disease
	The mechanism of action for various phosphorus-binding agents
Metabolism	**Metabolism**
The functions of phosphorus	Metabolic alterations to the calcium–phosphorus ratio with altered renal function, including phosphorus elevation as a compensatory mechanism for phosphorus excretion
The optimal calcium–phosphorus ratio	
The phosphorus content of body fluids	
	Glomerular filtration rate as an indicator of phosphorus tolerance
	The effect of parathyroid hormone in renal disease
	Renal osteodystrophy
Excretion	**Excretion**
Normal phosphorus excretion	Changes in phosphorus excretion with renal disease
	Phosphorus removal with dialysis

metabolism alone is insufficient to meet the challenges inherent in the clinical setting. In **Exhibit 7–2,** an advanced practice dietitian describes in very simple terms how she thinks of nutrition pathophysiology for patients with COPD.

Nutrition Pathophysiology: A Summary

Advanced practice dietitians have learned more than the rote clinical application of the forms, formulas, and dietetics tradition to direct patient care; they also understand the nutrition pathology of disease and apply this knowledge directly to the care of individual patients. Knowledge and skill in nutrition pathophysiology form the basis of nutrition intervention and MNT. A clear understanding of the role of nutrition in the pathology of disease provides the basis to develop the most effective nutritional interventions.

Table 7–3 A Proposed Outline for a Graduate-Level Nutrition Pathophysiology Course

---

Concepts in Nutrition Pathophysiology

A Brief Review of Cellular Metabolism

Nutrition Pathophysiology Related to Foodborne Illness

    Pesticides, Irradiated Foods, Additives, and Allergens

    Foodborne and Waterborne Illness

Nutrition Pathophysiology Related to Inadequate Food and Nutrient Intake

    Malnutrition and Starvation

    Anemia

    Osteoporosis

Nutrition Pathophysiology Related to Excessive Food and Nutrient Intake

    Obesity

    Diabetes

    Heart Disease

    Liver Disease

    Renal Disease

Nutrition Pathophysiology of Injury

    Injury, Wounds, and Healing

    Inflammation and Barriers to Inflammation, Infection, and Sepsis

    AIDS

    Tumerogenesis and Neoplasia

Nutrition Pathophysiology of Organ-Specific Disease

    Pulmonary Disease

    Gastrointestinal Disease

ADVANCED MEDICAL NUTRITION THERAPY

"No disease that can be treated by diet should be treated with any other means."
—Maimonides[29]

MNT is provided under the aegis of the four-step Nutrition Care Process, in which the advanced practice dietitian (1) performs a nutrition assessment, (2) makes a nutrition diagnosis, (3) provides a nutrition intervention, and (4) performs nutrition monitoring and evaluation. The nutrition intervention provided by the advanced practice dietitian is based on the best available evidence but is individualized to the patient and his or her circumstances so as to obtain the maximum therapeutic effect.

EXHIBIT 7–2

Advanced Practice with Patients Who Have Chronic Obstructive Pulmonary Disease

As an advanced practice dietitian, I'm expected to do research and to publish. I might have an abstract for the ADA meeting, or I might put something in our physician newsletter. That's one of the requirements.

Where I used my advanced practice skills was in the respiratory care unit. With those patients, it was so important that they weren't overfed—but I think everyone knows about that. The other thing I did was spend a lot of time correcting electrolytes, especially magnesium and phosphorus. Phosphorus plays such a big role in breathing. It enhances the release of oxygen from hemoglobin and is used in muscle function. Correcting electrolytes is something that basic level dietitians wouldn't do. They would focus on calories, protein, albumin, transferrin levels. They wouldn't take the time to look at electrolytes.

Of course, with COPD patients, you also have to know quite a bit about blood gases, including what the numbers mean and what is an expected CO_2 level in the arterial blood. In addition, you have to know quite a bit about lung function. For example, to use the Swinamer equation, you need to have the tidal volume, and you need to talk with the respiratory therapist to know what tidal volume means. You need to know the respiratory rate, including what is normal versus what is fast or slow; you need to know about gas exchange and the function of the intercostal muscles.

Another issue is following the patients daily. Now that I do that, I wish I would always have had time to see patients every day.

The basic level practitioner will insist on rules for MNT and will likely provide the same or very similar therapy to all patients with the same category of disease—for example, providing a diet that is low in saturated fat to all patients with heart disease, or using the same method of teaching a diabetic diet. In contrast, the advanced practice dietitian uses diagnostic reasoning skills to identify a nutrition diagnosis based on complex and detailed patient information about the patient rather than the disease. Such a professional may refer to guidelines for MNT, but adapts them as needed to reflect the situation at hand. Although the advanced practice dietitian is comfortable with the most complex of nutrition interventions, he or she typically individualizes and simplifies those strategies to obtain maximum results.

As expected, some of the advanced practice dietitians in our study demonstrated expertise in specialized areas. They easily discussed complex therapy and difficult patients, spontaneously giving rich examples of sophisticated interventions. These examples were peppered with comments about the importance of knowing more than "just what's in the book." Rather than a single approach, they depended on their experience and knowledge to select from a wide variety of interventions those that would produce the best result for the patient.

These dietitians referred to current literature and to current guidelines to guide—but not replace—their thinking. They did not quote specific formulas or slogans, but were eager to entertain difficult opinions or to participate in debate. They thoughtfully reviewed patient data and the treatment plan, and asked thought-provoking questions. The novice knows one disease and one treatment for it. By contrast, the expert intimately understands the nuances of the disease and knows several effective treatments for it (as well as the ineffective ones). The expert knows the indications, the contraindications, and the implications of comorbidities and is well versed in how to achieve the desired outcomes in a variety of ways with a variety of patients.

One participant in our study defined advanced practice as follows:

> When they come with that complex problem, you don't stop and think, "Well, how will I know?" They talk to you, and you can just start quoting the literature, you can talk to them about what's going on, and you can look at the patient and help figure something out. Maybe you can't fix it, but you realize where your limitations are and where your potential is.

This quote demonstrates the confidence in his or her expertise possessed by the advanced practice dietitian, along with the dietitian's acknowledgment of the limitations of that expertise.

Advanced practice dietitians are reluctant to perform outside their area of expertise because they are uncomfortable in assuming a less than an expert role. While sometimes perceived as inflexibility, this trait really typifies their commitment to expert performance. Participants demonstrate their true flexibility by quickly learning and adapting new technology or information to advance their own practice.

Table 7–4 illustrates the progression from knowledge to expertise along a continuum. Although this table refers to potassium, a similar table could readily be developed for other topics. For example, renal and nutrition support dietitians will experience a similar knowledge progression for sodium, phosphorus, magnesium, and other electrolytes. Dietitians working with diabetes and obesity could develop a continuum of knowledge related to counseling skills.

Advanced practice in MNT practice is not typically based on textbooks or diet manuals, but rather on data from primary literature sources. The advanced practice dietitians who participated in our study mentioned regularly reading peer-reviewed

Table 7–4 The Progression of Knowledge and Skill Along the Potassium Continuum

Level of Practice	Knowledge and Skill
Technician	The DRI for potassium is 4700 mg/day for an adult; normal serum values are 3.5–5.5 mEq/L. The technician can find values for children or other age groups. He or she can convert potassium from milligrams into milliequivalents, and back into milligrams.
General/basic	The generalist knows that there are cardiac effects with hyperkalemia and that delayed gastric emptying can occur with hypokalemia. The generalist also knows many high- and low-potassium foods and may recognize the standard dose for potassium replacement.
Specialist	The specialist knows that, as a general rule, serum potassium levels change by 0.1 mEq/dL with a 10 mEq change in intake. He or she also knows that this rule usually works well to manipulate serum levels within the normal range. The specialist can anticipate how serum potassium levels will change in concert with rising creatinine levels, diarrhea, surgery, postoperative diuresis, and other common clinical conditions. The specialist can also anticipate changes in serum potassium in response to furosemide, aldactone, or amphotericin administration. He or she may spend time calculating hourly potassium rates and thinking about how much potassium the patient has received since a bag of parenteral nutrition was hung or the blood was drawn. The specialist knows how to respond to an inadequate or excessive potassium dose.
Advanced	The advanced practice dietitian has internalized the information possessed by lower-level practitioners, but is not often called on to quote it. The advanced practice dietitian works with less detail, but knows instantly if a suggested change in potassium intake is likely to achieve the desired result. When faced with the need to increase or decrease potassium intake, the advanced practice dietitian provides a range of acceptable intake rather than a single number. He or she may ask about the desired serum potassium value, and then order the potassium dose to achieve that level. The advanced practice dietitian may focus on patients or groups of patients who develop hypokalemia or hyperkalemia, and create interventions that prevent these complications. The advanced practice dietitian provides individualized care, but also focuses on the system level.

nutrition-focused journals such as *Journal of the American Dietetic Association, American Journal of Clinical Nutrition, Journal of Renal Nutrition,* and *Journal of Parenteral and Enteral Nutrition.* Several also mentioned receiving electronic copies of the table of contents of *New England Journal of Medicine* and *Journal of the American Medical Association* as part of their effort to remain current with medical issues. Others reported reading specialty journals such as *Pediatrics, Gastroenterology, Critical Care Medicine,* or *Bariatric Surgery,* which allowed them to keep abreast of nutrition-related articles being read by their physician colleagues.

The advanced practice dietitians in our study were distinguished by their reading habits. Most read newsletters from several specialty practice areas, but recognized that these publications were of variable quality. They spent more time with the higher-quality, peer-reviewed publications and less time with the editor-reviewed, practice-oriented magazines and newsletters. They had developed refined literature search and evidence analysis skills. In addition, they were able to judge the quality of research articles and critique (rather than criticize) research.

Experienced dietitians have clearly asked for more information about MNT. With the volume of emerging literature increasing each year, it seems appropriate to offer graduate-level courses that teach dietitians how to review emerging MNT information and apply it to practice; **Table 7–5** outlines the topics that might be covered in such a course. While this approach is introduced in basic level practice, dietitians at the advanced level must be expert at reading practice-based literature, judging its quality, and incorporating its lessons into their everyday practice.

NUTRITION COUNSELING

"Tell me what you eat, and I will tell you what you are." —Jean Anthelme Brillat-Savarin[30]

Counseling may be defined as professional guidance of an individual via psychological methods, especially the collection of case history data through the use of techniques including personal interviews and testing of interests and aptitudes.[8] *Nutrition counseling* has been defined as "a supportive process, characterized by a collaborative counselor–patient/client relationship, to set priorities, establish goals, and create individualized action plans that acknowledge and foster responsibility for self-care to treat an existing condition and promote health."[31]

Table 7–5 Suggested Topics for a Graduate-Level Course in Advanced Medical Nutrition Therapy

Advanced Medical Nutrition Therapy
Introduction to Evidence-Based Medical Nutrition Therapy
    Literature-Searching Techniques
    Evaluating Literature Quality
    Guidelines and Guideline Development
Nutrition Intervention: Intake of Foods, Meals, and Snacks
    Evaluating the Quality of Emerging Food and Nutrition Information
    Evaluating the Quality of Food and Nutrient Allergy Information
    Using the Nutrition History and Physical Exam to Identify Altered Intake
        General Appearance and Examination of the Skin
        Chewing and Swallowing
        Range of Motion and Other Physical Limitations
        The Abdominal Exam
    Co-morbidities and Impaired Intake
        Depression
        Eating Disorders
        Substance Abuse
Nutrition Intervention: Enteral and Parenteral Nutrition
    The Scientific Basis for Enteral and Parenteral Product Evaluation
    Prevention and Management of Enteral and Parenteral Complications
Nutrition Intervention: Medical Food, Vitamin and Mineral Supplements
    FDA Regulation of Foods, Nutrients, Supplements, and Drugs
Nutrition Intervention: Bioactive Supplements
Nutrition Intervention: Complementary and Alternative Therapy

In dietetics, the phrase "nutrition counseling" has often been substituted for "nutrition education" to increase the perceived importance of the nutrition education function. In truth, counseling and education are not synonymous. *Nutrition education* has been defined as "instruction or training intended to build or reinforce basic nutrition-related knowledge, or to provide essential nutrition-related information until the patient or client returns."[31] Both basic nutrition education and nutrition education that results in in-depth knowledge are described in the standardized language of dietetics.[31] Nutrition education may be delivered to a single patient, to a patient and his or her family members, or in a classroom setting.

Nutrition education encompasses the traditional activity of "teaching the patient about his or her diet" or "giving the patient a copy of his or her diet"—a task that is frequently performed in an acute care setting. Nutrition education implies a one-way delivery of information with the objective of increasing knowledge. This activity is usually performed in a single encounter during a short hospital stay. In some cases, the dietitian may have the opportunity to return or to schedule the patient for a clinic visit, but this is not always possible.

In contrast to nutrition education, nutrition counseling implies two-way communication between the dietitian and the patient/client. Also, incorporation of the word "process" into the definition of counseling implies an activity that takes place over an extended period of time rather than in a single episode. In particular, nutrition counseling begins with a detailed assessment in which the dietitian may spend several sessions actively listening to the client. The purpose of these sessions is to aid both dietitian and client in creating achievable, measurable goals for behavior change and then measuring progress toward those outcomes. Also, while dietitians most assuredly use their counseling skills to foster changes in eating and other health behaviors, they also apply their counseling skills to their interactions with physicians, caregivers, nurses, or other providers.

According to one advanced practice dietitian with expertise in counseling:

> The basic level dietitian gives standardized information and rarely tailors the intervention to the patient. The philosophy of the basic level dietitian is "I have a goal for you. This is what you need to do." This method of dealing with dietary change leads to one or two visits, but no continuity and not much long-term behavior change. Most dietitians do not know what to do if clients come more than twice because they have run out of information to hand them.

Another advanced practice dietitian commented:

> You know they [basic level dietitians] might know the transtheoretical model. But whether or not they've actually been able to apply it in terms of the key messages they provide to the patient, or the materials or types of goals they set with the individual, that's a different thing.

Various attempts to understand not only behavior, but also ways to change that behavior, have resulted in the emergence of numerous counseling theories. These theories, which were initially developed by psychologists and psychiatrists, have been applied to nutrition and lifestyle issues to improve adherence to recommendations and improve health outcomes. Counseling is a well-established field that encompasses a broad knowledgebase. Professionals who use the title of "Counselor" typically have an advanced degree in some aspect of psychology, obtain supervised practice experience in the application of counseling skills, and pass a certifying exam. They may also belong to a professional organization for counselors.

Nutrition counseling incorporates two components: advanced MNT skills (as discussed in the previous section in this chapter) and advanced counseling skills needed to foster patient adherence to nutrition intervention. Thus dietitians often take counseling courses as part of a graduate-level nutrition program. Some dietitians apply these counseling skills in practice to engender improved nutritional outcomes for patients or clients. Others use their counseling skills to negotiate the details of nutrition intervention with physicians, nurses, or other providers. Dietitians who participate in research may apply their counseling skills to improve protocol adherence in clinical trials. Dietitians may also use their counseling skills in an effort to work more effectively with colleagues and support staff. Thus it is proposed that the advanced practice dietitian has expertise in one or more of the counseling models that are described next.

Cognitive-Behavioral Theory

Cognitive-behavioral theory is based on the idea that all behavior is learned. To change a behavior, therefore, the therapist identifies the details of the problem behavior that precipitate events resulting in the target behavior. This knowledge of the reasons for problem behavior is then used to develop an intervention. The therapist works with the client to develop a strategy that changes the behavior by restructuring either the behavior or the thinking that underlies the behavior.[32] Restructured behavior, in turn, enhances adherence.

The behavioral portion of cognitive-behavioral therapy provides patients with principles and techniques to use in modifying their eating and exercise behaviors. Behavioral therapy does not depend on an understanding of the behavior, but rather seeks to modify behavior using techniques such as goal setting and stimulus control. The cognitive portion of cognitive-behavioral therapy then adds problem-solving and cognitive-restructuring techniques to the behavioral approach.[32]

Health Belief Model

The health belief model is a psychological model that seeks to explain and predict health-related behaviors by focusing on an individual's attitudes and beliefs. It provides a framework to understand health behaviors in terms of the individual's perceived susceptibility, perceived severity, perceived benefits, perceived barriers, and self-efficacy relative to a particular health outcome.[33] The health belief model is based on the assumption that an individual will be motivated to take health-related action if that person can avoid or manage a negative health condition (e.g., hypertension) or has an expectation that by taking a recommended action, a negative health condition can be avoided (e.g., decreasing intake of high-sodium foods will help prevent stroke). The patient must also believe that he or she can successfully perform the health action (e.g., I can reduce my intake of fried foods). The health belief model has been applied by dietitians in osteoporosis prevention, for example.[34]

Social Learning Theory

Social learning theory, also known as social cognitive theory, provides a framework for understanding, predicting, and changing behavior.[35] This theory identifies a dynamic, reciprocal relationship between the environment, the person, and his or her behavior. The person can be both an agent for change and a responder to change. Social cognitive theory emphasizes the importance of observing and modeling the behaviors, attitudes, and emotional reactions of others. Determinants of behavior include goals, outcome expectations, and self-efficacy. Reinforcements either increase or decrease the likelihood that the behavior will be repeated. This model has been applied by dietitians in changing behavior—for example, to reduce a patient's risk of a second primary cancer and to increase fruit and vegetable intake in school-aged children.[36–38]

Transtheoretical Model

One of the counseling models familiar to dietitians is the transtheoretical model (also known as the stages of change model), which was developed by Prochaska.[39] This model involves identifying patients' thinking in response to achieving health-related goals. Patients are categorized as being in one of five stages of change: precontemplation, contemplation, preparation, action, and maintenance. Using the transtheoretical model, the dietitian discerns which stage of change is most reflective of the patient's status relative to the desired food and nutrition goals and then develops a strategy intended to move the patient farther along the path toward the desired behavior change.[40]

Nutrition Counseling: A Summary

The models mentioned in this section are ones that are commonly used to counsel patients to change their food- and nutrition-related behavior. Some are more complex than others, and some may be preferred by experienced nutrition counselors. Developing the ability to use these models and the accompanying strategies effectively, and being able to individualize them to the needs of a particular client, requires not only study but also practice in the clinical setting. To develop advanced practice counseling skills, dietitians must have extensive practice experience. **Table 7–6** provides suggested topics for a course in nutrition counseling while **Exhibit 7–3** provides insight into how an advanced practice dietitian might interact with a client.

Table 7-6 A Proposed Outline for a Graduate-Level Course in Nutrition Counseling

The Theoretical Basis for Counseling
Counseling Theories
   Cognitive-Behavioral Theory
   Health Belief Model
   Social Learning Theory
   Transtheoretical Model
Developing and Implementing Counseling Strategies
   Cognitive Restructuring
   Goal Setting
   Motivational Interviewing
   Problem Solving
   Rewards/Contingency Management
   Self-Monitoring
   Social Support
   Stimulus Control
   Stress Management
Counseling Practicum: Mentored practice with all models and strategies for four hours per week for 15 weeks

EXHIBIT 7-3

Active Listening as the Basis for Intervention

We're doing one project now where we counsel obese patients who have failed other programs. Our program runs for nine sessions. We spend the first two or three sessions just doing active listening. We try to find out how the person is feeling about the whole process. We try to find out what may have worked for him or her in the past. We take the time to understand, rather than just giving information. We do this before we come up with a diagnosis, because if you take the time up front, you can be more successful. With a careful assessment, the advanced practice dietitian counselor can carefully tailor the intervention and knows when to give information at a time when the patient is ready to make a change.

NUTRITION OUTCOMES RESEARCH

"There are, in fact, two things: science and opinion; the former begets knowledge, the latter ignorance." —*Hippocrates*[6]

Outcomes research has been defined as "the rigorous determination of what works in medical care and what does not."[41] Its purpose is to help patients, providers, payers, administrators, and clinicians make informed choices, especially as related to interventions.[42] Outcomes research is a relatively new research method whose development represents an outgrowth of the economic restrictions associated with increased healthcare costs. As managed care organizations began to compete based on the results obtained by clinicians working in their organizations, they recognized the need to demonstrate treatment efficiency. At the same time, wide variations in patterns of care across different geographic locations were found to be the norm. To determine which healthcare services were most beneficial, outcomes research was developed and quickly evolved into an important means to help patients, providers, payers, administrators, and clinicians make informed choices.

According to the Agency for Healthcare Research and Quality, outcomes research seeks to understand the end results of particular healthcare practices and interventions. End results include effects that people experience and care about, such as change in the ability to function. In particular, for individuals with chronic conditions—where cure is not always possible—end results include both quality of life and mortality. By linking the care people get to the outcomes they experience, outcomes research has become the key to developing better ways to monitor and improve the quality of care. Supporting improvements in health outcomes is a strategic goal of the Agency for Healthcare Research and Quality.[43]

One of the defining characteristics of any profession is the unique body of knowledge and practices that members of the profession deploy. In the health professions, research is used to support and expand the knowledge that serves as the foundation of dietetics. Research is also used to develop and measure treatment effectiveness. This research function is crucial to justify payment for services. In addition, research findings expand the body of knowledge that is taught to succeeding generations of practitioners. Research findings guide us as to what works and helps us to decide which practices can be discarded. As aptly stated in a 1997 editorial in *Journal of the American Dietetic Association*, research is the scientific underpinning of the dietetics profession.[44]

Like most healthcare professions, dietetics has evolved from having its roots in pragmatism, tradition, and the personal preferences of a few influential individuals to an intervention-oriented, science-based profession. Dietitians have used bits and pieces of findings from basic nutrition science, ferreted out isolated facts from medicine and nursing, applied epidemiologic findings, and observed their own experience to develop patient-specific interventions and monitoring. However, this process is not truly research. Rather, research comprises the systematic application of a structured scientific process to a specific problem.

Nutrition scientists, nurses, physicians, and epidemiologists all have their own agendas when it comes to research. Some of these investigators conduct studies that are of interest to dietitians. Nevertheless, the basic nutrition science, nursing, physician, or epidemiology research agenda is not designed to support the advancement of dietetics. Examples of the types of research questions that dietitians need to answer for the field to move forward are included within ADA's research agenda, which is shown in **Table 7–7.** To effectively advance dietetics research, we

---

Table 7–7 Suggested Medical Nutrition Therapy Research Topics Associated with the American Dietetic Association's Research Priorities[45]

Prevention and Treatment of Obesity and Associated Chronic Diseases
· Which infant feeding practices are associated with higher incidence of childhood obesity?
· Is there a relationship between the timing of food intake and weight gain or loss?

Effective Nutrition and Lifestyle Change Interventions
· What are the most effective strategies to improve dietary adherence?
· Which nutrients or combinations of nutrients are most likely to require supplementation in specific diseases?

Translation of Research into Nutrition Interventions and Programs
· How should development and testing of nutrition interventions based on basic science research proceed?
· Which nutrition programs might be most effective in reducing specific nutrition or medical diagnoses?

Effective Nutrition Indicators and Outcome Measures
· Can biomarkers be developed for specific nutrition diagnoses?
· Which outcome measures are easiest to apply to resolution of nutrition diagnoses?

Dietetics Education and Retention
· What is needed to increase career satisfaction for dietitians?
· What are the best methods to distribute new knowledge and skills to experienced dietitians?

(continues)

Table 7–7 Continued

Delivery of and Payment for Dietetic Services

· What is the optimal duration and timing of nutritional interventions for specific nutrition diagnoses?

· What healthcare cost reductions are associated with medical nutrition therapy provided by a registered dietitian?

Customer Satisfaction

· What are the most effective measures of customer satisfaction with medical nutrition therapy?

· Which strategies should dietitians use to increase referrals and utilization of medical nutrition therapy?

Nutrients and Gene Expression

· Which preventive strategies can be implemented for individuals and populations with a genetic propensity to develop certain diseases?

· How effective are preventive strategies in delaying or ameliorating the impact of a genetic propensity to develop specific diseases?

---

will need trained researchers who can successfully obtain funding for dietetics research. This need is a primary reason to develop additional graduate programs and terminal degrees in dietetics.

The advanced practice dietitians who participated in our study clearly recognized the importance of research. They incorporated research findings into practice, but also read and critiqued research studies. According to several of these dietitians, the ability to fluently quote the literature relevant to practice was a mandatory skill required to garner respect in the clinical setting. However, several of the dietitians had taken their interest in research a step further, by generating research questions and participating in studies with their colleagues. Others had participated in research studies, and one or two clinicians had served as principal investigators. Several mentioned the need to answer practice-based questions as key considerations in nutrition research. Others focused on the need for access to students who could help with practice-based research projects.

One participant in our study was particularly optimistic about doing research:

> I know that some of the big researchers say that if you don't have that National Institutes of Health money, you're pretty much out of luck. But I really and truly think that if we would use good common sense and some of our practice group research dollars, it is possible to do the work that needs to be done. You can certainly work on outcomes, especially now that we'll have nutrition diagnostic language to describe what is done. You can then collect and aggregate data.

Other advanced practice dietitians had initiated projects intended to capture performance improvement data. Some had worked with colleagues in their facility or with members of their practice group to develop research projects. Clearly, these advanced practice dietitians valued the research process and research findings supporting practice. One described her experience in a huge multicenter trial in **Exhibit 7–4.**

Entry-level dietitians must be competent to interpret and incorporate new scientific knowledge into practice.[46] Nevertheless, there is no mandate to train basic level dietitians to judge the quality of research studies, to generate new scientific knowledge, or to measure the outcomes of therapy. Increasingly, research opportunities are reserved for investigators with doctoral-level preparation who have postdoctoral training in research methodology. Even so, some authors insist that research opportunities and output of dietitians have not been optimized.[47] Although research is typically a component of master's degree programs, Schiller found that relatively few RDs were, in fact, trained to do research.[47] Eck described an outcomes research model and illustrated the value of outcomes research to clinical practice;[48] it is unknown whether Eck's model is in widespread use. Dietitians anecdotally state that they are not interested in doing research, but their interest in research might potentially increase if more clinically relevant research projects were developed.[49]

Dietitians could very likely learn from the experiences of the physical therapy and nursing professions. When they implemented graduate degrees as a prerequisite for entry-level practice, the students entering the profession were required to do research projects. As a result of their efforts, the physical therapy profession has

EXHIBIT 7–4

A Research Opportunity

Research is important. Even though I was in a clinical outpatient setting, I was still doing research. I didn't get paid to do the NIH hemodialysis study, but I did it in my free time. It was fantastic—one of the best experiences I've had. It gave me ongoing research training. I got to participate in these large NIH meetings. I got to meet with all these creative people with all their fantastic ideas. Sometimes people think, "Well, I'm not getting paid for this, so I'm not going to do it." But that's crazy! They just don't know how valuable it is to have that experience.

accumulated large amounts of practice-based data justifying reimbursement for physical therapy services. In nursing, advanced practice nursing research methods courses focus on outcomes research rather than traditional experimental designs. The results of research conducted by advanced practice nursing students are used to develop and test nursing interventions and to justify the role of the advanced practice nurse. Because they learned outcomes research methods as part of their graduate education, physical therapists and advanced practice nurses have the skills needed to further define and expand their practice. These skills can be used in an ongoing fashion to justify advancement to higher-level positions and document effectiveness of care. As a result, the nursing literature is full of studies documenting that advanced practice nurses decrease the length of hospital stays, readmission rates, and costs as well as provide more efficient coordination of services.[50]

To date, members of the dietetics profession have shown at least some interest in conducting outcomes research studies. For example, one study has demonstrated the positive impact of dietitian-implemented nutrition guidelines on pregnancy outcomes for pregnant women with diabetes.[51] Other studies have identified positive outcomes with nutrition interventions in heart failure and prevention of unintentional weight loss in residential healthcare facilities.[52,53] These and other subsequent studies will no doubt be incorporated into the professional body of knowledge and justify the need for MNT going forward. It is anticipated that one role for the advanced practice dietitian will be to identify those areas where studies are needed and to collaborate with researchers to conduct the appropriate studies.

The dietetics profession can clearly benefit from outcomes research related to the practice of MNT. Outcomes research can help to test and refine developing nutrition interventions. It can also benefit the profession by demonstrating the need for MNT for specific diseases and conditions. In addition, outcomes research will help us to identify what does not work, thereby allowing us to discard unnecessary practices and focus on the effective ones. Finally, outcomes research can help us focus on our own practice and better define and expand what we do.

SUMMARY

This chapter explored the basis of expertise for practitioners of MNT. The body of knowledge supporting MNT continues to increase each month. Already, there is sufficient information to launch several graduate-level courses directly related to advanced MNT. This chapter provided a brief overview of this coursework, including topic outlines and suggestions for graduate-level courses in MNT. The purpose of these courses should be to provide information in sufficient depth to allow dietitians to function at an expert level in the clinical environment. Topics covered should include nutrition pharmacology, nutrition physiology, advanced MNT, counseling, and outcomes research. Educators may use this information to initiate course development, expanding it with detail from the current literature.

KEY POINTS

- The profession of dietetics has not delineated the educational content for programs leading to advanced MNT practice. We need to distinguish between basic and advanced MNT knowledge and skills and then develop educational programs to meet the needs of both levels of practice.
- Among participants in our study, nutrition pharmacology was the most frequently mentioned area of expertise required for advanced practice dietitians in MNT. A significant role awaits dietitians in nutrition pharmacology, and a large body of knowledge for study and application to practice already exists.
- The focus of nutrition teaching and research has traditionally been normal nutrition, nutrition education, or nutrition epidemiology. These areas are of interest academically, but expansion of the educational agenda into nutrition pathophysiology and the nutritional treatment of disease is needed. Advanced practice dietitians have identified some of these areas of practice, but further research is needed to support advanced dietetics practice.
- MNT is taught as part of preparation for basic level dietetics practice. Unfortunately, there is rarely sufficient time within a generalist dietetics program to cover current research and evolving issues in advanced MNT practice.
- The advanced practice dietitian who works with patients who must modify their lifestyle to improve their health must possesses advanced counseling skills. Such skills enable the dietitian to identify the etiologies of complex nutrition problems and devise the patient-centered strategies most likely to achieve successful behavior change.
- The advanced practice dietitian possesses sufficient outcomes research skills to design outcomes studies that not merely justify, but also advance, practice.

SUGGESTED READING

Nutrition Pharmacology

AHFS drug information. Bethesda, MD: American Hospital Formulary Service, 2005.

DiPiro JT, Talbert RL, Ye, GC, Matzke GR, Wells BG, Posey LM. *Pharmacotherapy.* New York: McGraw-Hill, 2002.

Drug facts and comparisons. St. Louis: Walters Klewer, 2005.

Laurence BL, Lazo J, Parker K (eds.). *Goodman and Gilman's pharmacologic basis of therapeutics.* New York: McGraw-Hill, 2005.

McCabe BJ, Frankel EH, Wolfe JJ (eds.). *Handbook of food and drug interactions.* Boca Raton: CRC, 2003.

Nutrition Pathophysiology

ACP Journal Club. Available by subscription only at http://www.acpjc.org/.

This site contains critiques of clinical trials.

Agency for Healthcare Research and Quality. National guideline clearinghouse. Available at http://guidelines.gov/.

This evidence-based practice website provides an opportunity for organizations to post guidelines for managing various diseases and conditions. It contains a number of guidelines relevant to nutrition.

American Dietetic Association. Evidence analysis library. Available at www.adaevidencelibrary .com/.

This site contains expert analysis of the literature on dozens of questions of interest to dietitians. It is available free of charge to ADA members.

Bowman BA, Russell RM (eds.). *Present knowledge in nutrition,* 9th ed. Washington, DC: International Life Sciences Institute, 2006.

Cochrane Library. Available at http://www3.interscience.wiley.com/cgi-bin/mrwhome/ 106568753/HOME.

This British library of evidence analysis projects contains the results of dozens of projects related to medical nutrition therapy.

Shils ME, Shike M, Ross AC, Caballero B, Cousins RJ. *Modern nutrition in health and disease,* 10th ed. Philadelphia: Lippincott Williams and Wilkins, 2005.

Nutrition Counseling

Bandura A. *Social foundations of thought and action: A social cognitive theory.* Englewood Cliffs, NJ: Prentice Hall, 1985.

International Listening Organization. Available at http://www.listen.org/Templates/welcome .htm.

This organization provides education to members interested in the value of listening.

Prochaska JO, Norcross JC. *Systems of psychotherapy: A transtheoretical analysis,* 4th ed. Belmont, CA: Wadsworth, 2002.

Snetselaar L. *Nutrition counseling in lifestyle change.* New York: CRC Press, 2006.

Snetselaar L. *Nutrition counseling skills: Assessment, treatment, and evaluation.* Boston: Jones and Bartlett, 2002.

Outcomes Research

Ireton-Jones CS, Gottschlich MM, Bell SJ (eds.). *Practice-oriented nutrition research: An outcomes measurement approach.* Gaithersburg, MD: Aspen, 1998.

This text serves as an introduction to outcomes research with a focus on nutrition support topics.

Kane RL. *Understanding health care outcomes research.* Boston: Jones and Bartlett, 2004.

A text that applies to the broader healthcare environment.

Splett PL. *Outcomes research and economic analysis in research: Successful approaches.* In Monsen EL (ed.). Research Chicago: American Dietetic Association, 2003.

A brief chapter written by the most published outcomes researcher in dietetics.

User's guide to the medical literature: Essentials of evidence based practice. Chicago: American Medical Association, 2001.

This text is a compilation of articles that originally appeared in the *Journal of the American Medical Association.* The articles offer insights into interpreting and applying research in practice.

EXPERIENCES TO TRY

Nutrition Pharmacology

1. Graduate-level courses in pharmacology may be available online through colleges of nursing, medicine, or pharmacy. In some instances, enrollment is limited to those admitted to a specific program; in others, qualified graduate students from all areas are accepted. Consider enrolling in a course that offers an overview of pharmacology so that you can learn the drug classes, naming conventions. and mechanisms of action.

2. Make a list of the most commonly prescribed drugs in your particular area of practice. Make a chart that gives the indications and contraindications for the drug, the mechanism of action, and the side effects that might affect nutrient intake. Obtain this information from the package insert, *Physician's Desk Reference,* and the American Hospital Formulary Service. Compare your findings. Note the recommended course of treatment (amount and duration). Do the patients in your practice who take the drug exhibit the symptoms listed on the package insert? How many of them do and how many of them do not? Do the symptoms clear up if the patients

stop taking the drug? Can you design a nutrition intervention that modifies the response to the drug therapy?

3. Obtain the following articles:

> Dickerson RN, Roth-Yousey L. Medication effects on metabolic rate: A systematic review (Part 1). *Journal of the American Dietetic Association* 2005;105:835–843.

> Dickerson RN, Roth-Yousey L. Medication effects on metabolic rate: A systematic review (Part 2). *Journal of the American Dietetic Association* 2005;105:1002–1009.

After reading the articles, select one or two drugs that you commonly see in your practice. Conduct a literature search according to the methods the authors used and obtain articles that appeared after their review was published. Select the three articles that are most relevant to your area of practice. Read and grade them according to the methods used by the authors.

Nutrition Pathophysiology

1. Identify a disease with a strong nutritional component, but not one with which you are familiar. Find a medical pathophysiology textbook. Trace the pathology of the disease using the intake–absorption–metabolism–excretion model. Create a chart similar to the one in Exhibit 7–3.

Advanced Medical Nutrition Therapy

1. Arrange to interview a leading clinician in your area of practice. Formulate the questions in advance and share them with the leading clinician a week prior to the interview to give the interviewee time for reflection. Ask about which interventions the clinician uses, including which ones work, which ones don't work, and why. Ask how the clinician might have changed the interventions he or she uses over time. Take careful notes.

   After the interview, set aside some time to reflect on your own experience. Compare and contrast your experience to that of the leading clinician. Think about how the clinician's experience compares to that in the published literature. Briefly summarize your findings. Finally, think about which questions remain.

2. Select a current issue in MNT. Prepare a practice paper that follows this format: In the introduction, define and describe the issue, including its prevalence, incidence, and economic impact on society. In the body of the paper, describe at least two MNT interventions, including the rationale for each, and summarizing the differences of opinion about the interventions. Present a discussion of the relevant research that incorporates at least three

peer-reviewed research papers on each of the interventions. Finally, present a clear, concise argument for applying (or not applying) both interventions to specific patient populations.

3. Gather half a dozen nutrition-related journals, magazines, and newsletters. Spend a few minutes reading each one. Make notes as you read. Begin to compare the quality of the information. Is it authoritative? Well referenced? Based in sound scientific methods? Do you like or dislike the information because it agrees or disagrees with your viewpoint? Is the material challenging to understand? Compare what you find in journals with the nutrition information found on the National Institutes of Health website. What are your impressions? Can you establish a hierarchy of quality for the information? Is some information suitable for patients? For dietitians? For physicians?

Nutrition Counseling

1. At the end of the day, take a few minutes to reflect on the last counseling session you conducted. Did you use one of the models described in the text? One of the strategies? Would another model or strategy have worked better with that patient? Could you have uncovered additional information that might have helped shape your intervention? Can you imagine taking two or three sessions to uncover the patient's underlying issues? What questions would you ask in such a case?

2. Read about one of the counseling models or strategies that is unfamiliar to you. Devise a scenario where you would find that technique helpful. Introduce the new model or strategy into your practice. Try it on several patients. If you are not in a position to use it with patients, apply it to your interactions with your colleagues, your spouse, or your children. After a week, reflect on how well the model or strategy works for you. Is it comfortable? Did it improve your results?

Outcomes Research

1. New guidelines are released almost every month through the American Dietetic Association's Evidence Analysis Library (www.eatright.org). Select a topic of interest and read the guidelines for it. Note the strength of the evidence supporting the recommendations. Find an area where the evidence is not as strong as it could be. Develop an outline for an outcomes study that could be conducted in your practice. Contact a researcher with expertise

in that area of practice or one of the members of the oversight committee for the evidence analysis project. Arrange to discuss your question with that person. Does the question have merit? Think about how you might conduct a study. Could you collect data in your own practice? Could you collaborate with others who have similar interests?

2. Join the Dietetics Practice Based Research Network (www.eatright.org). This opportunity is available through the American Dietetic Association's website. Fill out the descriptive questionnaire, and review the projects. Would your question from exercise 1 be suitable for this group?

REFERENCES

1. Anatoli Boukreev. Brainy Quote Available at: http://www.brainyquote.com/quotes/quotes/a/anatolibou315912.html. Accessed August 21, 2007.

2. Smith RE, Patrick S, Michael P, Hager M. Medical nutrition therapy: The core of ADA's advocacy efforts (Part 1). *Journal of the American Dietetic Association* 2005; 105(5):825–834.

3. Lacey K, Pritchett E. Nutrition Care Process and Model: ADA adopts road map to quality care and outcomes management. *Journal of the American Dietetic Association* 2003;103(8):1061–1071.

4. Skipper A, Lewis NM. Using initiative to achieve autonomy: A model for advanced medical nutrition therapy practice. *Journal of the American Dietetic Association* 2006; 106(8):1219–1225.

5. Skipper A, Lewis NM. Clinical dietitians, employers, and educators are interested in advanced practice education and professional doctorate degrees in clinical nutrition. *Journal of the American Dietetic Association* 2006;106(12):2062–2066.

6. Hippocrates. *Wikiquote*. Available at http://en.wikiquote.org/wiki/Hippocrates. Accessed March 15, 2007.

7. Wikipedia. Available at http://www.wikipedia.org/. Accessed May 9, 2007.

8. Merriam-Webster Online. Available at www.m-w.com/. Accessed July 5, 2006.

9. Walton S, Cooksey JA, Knapp KK, Quist RM, Miller LM. Analysis of pharmacist and pharmacist-extender workforce in 1998–2000: Assessing predictors and differences across states. *Journal of the American Pharmacists Association* 2004;44(6):673–683.

10. Dickerson RN, Roth-Yousey L. Medication effects on metabolic rate: A systematic review (Part 2). *Journal of the American Dietetic Association* 2005;105(6):1002–1009.

11. Dickerson RN, Roth-Yousey L. Medication effects on metabolic rate: A systematic review (Part 1). *Journal of the American Dietetic Association* 2005;105(5):835–843.

12. Hager M, Hutchins A. Position of the American Dietetic Association: Integration of medical nutrition therapy and pharmacotherapy. *Journal of the American Dietetic Association* 2003;103(10):1361–1370.

13. Mueller CM, Colaizzo-Anas T, Shronts EP, Gaines JA. Order writing for parenteral nutrition by registered dietitians. *Journal of the American Dietetic Association* 1996;96(8): 764–768.

14. Olree K, Skipper A. The role of nutrition support dietitians as viewed by chief clinical and nutrition support dietitians: Implications for training. *Journal of the American Dietetic Association* 1997;97(12):1255–1260.

15. Wildish DE. An evidence-based approach for dietitian prescription of multiple vitamins and minerals. *Journal of the American Dietetic Association* 2004;104(5):779–786.

16. Green DM, Maillet JO, Touger-Decker R, Byham-Gray L, Matheson P. Functions performed by level of practice of registered dietitian members of the diabetes care and education dietetic practice group. *Journal of the American Dietetic Association* 2005; 105(8):1280–1284.

17. Shwide-Slavin C. Case study: A patient with type 1 diabetes who transitions to insulin pump therapy by working with an advanced practice dietitian. *Diabetes Spectrum* 2003; 16(1):37–40.

18. American Nurses Credentialing Center. Advanced diabetes management, dietitian version, board certification examination content outline. Available at http://www.diabetes educator.org/Certification/AdvClinicalDMOverview.shtml. Accessed March 13, 2007.

19. Wisdom quotes. Available at http://www.wisdomquotes.com/002629.html. Accessed April 17, 2007.

20. Cotran R, Kumar VTC. *Robbins pathologic basis of disease,* 6th ed. Philadelphia: W. B. Saunders, 1999.

21. *The State of Food Insecurity in the World 2005.* Rome: Food and Agriculture Organization of the United Nations, 2005.

22. Nord M. Fewer households had difficulty putting enough food on the table in 2005. In *Amber waves* (p. 1). Washington, DC: U.S. Department of Agriculture, 2007.

23. Skalicky A, Meyers A, Adams W, Yang Z, Cook J, Frank D. Child food insecurity and iron deficiency anemia in low-income infants and toddlers in the United States. *Maternal and Child Health* 2006;10(2):177–185.

24. Sullivan D, Bopp M, Roberson P. Protein-energy undernutrition and life-threatening complications among the hospitalized elderly. *Journal of General Internal Medicine* 2002;17(12):923–932.

25. Thomas DR, Zdrowski CD, Wilson M-M, et al. Malnutrition in subacute care. *American Journal of Clinical Nutrition* 2002;75(2):308–313.

26. Stover P. Influence of human genetic variation on nutritional requirements. *American Journal of Clinical Nutrition* 2006;83(2):436S–442S.

27. Loos RJ, Ruchat S, Rankinen T, Tremblay A, Perusse L, Bouchard C. Adiponectin and adiponectin receptor gene variants in relation to resting metabolic rate, respiratory quotient, and adiposity-related phenotypes in the Quebec Family Study. *American Journal of Clinical Nutrition* 2007;85(1):26–34.

28. Ordovas JM, Corella D, Cupples LA, et al. Polyunsaturated fatty acids modulate the effects of the APOA1 G-A polymorphism on HDL-cholesterol concentrations in a sex-specific manner: The Framingham Study. *American Journal of Clinical Nutrition* 2002;75(1):38–46.

29. Wikiquote. Available at http://en.wikiquote.org/wiki/Maimonides. Accessed March 15, 2007.

30. Brillat-Savarin J. The physiology of taste. Available at http://www.quotationspage .com/quotes/Anthelme_Brillat-Savarin/. Accessed May 10, 2007.

31. *Nutrition diagnosis and intervention: Standardized language for the nutrition care process.* Chicago: American Dietetic Association, 2006.

32. Fabricatore A. Behavior therapy and cognitive-behavior therapy of obesity: Is there a difference? *Journal of the American Dietetic Association* 2007;107(1):92–104.

33. Kloeblen AS. Folate knowledge, intake from fortified grain products, and periconceptional supplementation patterns of a sample of low-income pregnant women according to the health belief model. *Journal of the American Dietetic Association* 1999;99(1): 33–38.

34. Tussing L, Chapman-Novakofski K. Osteoporosis prevention education: Behavior theories and calcium intake. *Journal of the American Dietetic Association* 2005;105:92–97.

35. Bandura A. *Social learning theory.* Englewood Cliffs, NJ: Prentice Hall, 1977.

36. Mendoza M, Balvin L, Ramirez R, Mobley CC, Trevino RP. The Bienestar After School Health Club: A component of a school-based nutrition intervention program. *Journal of the American Dietetic Association* 1997;97(9):A72.

37. Falciglia G, Whittle K, Levin L, Steward D. A clinical-based intervention improves diet in patients with head and neck cancer at risk for second primary cancer. *Journal of the American Dietetic Association* 2005;105(10):1609–1612.

38. Gribble LS, Falciglia G, Davis AM, Couch SC. A curriculum based on social learning theory emphasizing fruit exposure and positive parent child-feeding strategies: A pilot study. *Journal of the American Dietetic Association* 2003;103(1):100–103.

39. Greene GW, Rossi SR, Rossi JS, Velicer WF, Fava JL, Prochaska JO. Dietary applications of the stages of change model. *Journal of the American Dietetic Association* 1999; 99(6):673–678.

40. Nothwehr F, Snetselaar L, Yang J, Wu H. Stage of change for healthful eating and use of behavioral strategies. *Journal of the American Dietetic Association* 2006;106(7): 1035–1041.

41. Ireton-Jones CS, Gottschlich M, Bell SE. *Practice-oriented nutrition research: An outcomes measurement approach.* Gaithersburg, MD: Aspen, 1998.

42. Epstein A. The outcomes movement: Will it get us where we want to go? *New England Journal of Medicine* 1990;323(4):266–270.

43. Agency for Healthcare Research and Quality. Outcomes research: Fact sheet. AHRQ Publication No. 00-P011. Available at http://www.ahrq.gov/clinic/outfact.htm. Accessed May 11, 2007.

44. Dwyer JT. Scientific underpinnings for the profession: Dietitians in research. *Journal of the American Dietetic Association* 1997;97(6):593–597.

45. Costellanos VH, Myers EF, Shanklin, CW. The ADAs research priorities contribute to a bright future for dietetics professionals. *Journal of the American Dietetic Association* 2004;104(4):678–680.

46. Bruening KS, Mitchell BE, Pfeiffer MM. 2002 accreditation standards for dietetics education. *Journal of the American Dietetic Association* 2002;102(4):566–577.

47. Schiller MR. Research activities and research skill needs of nutrition support dietitians. *Journal of the American Dietetic Association* 1988;88(9):345–346.

48. Eck LH, Slawson DL, Williams R, Smith K, Harmon-Clayton K, Oliver D. A model for making outcomes research standard practice in clinical dietetics. *Journal of the American Dietetic Association* 1998;98(4):451–457.

49. Slawson DL, Clemens LH. Research and the clinical dietitian: Perceptions of the research process and preferred routes to obtaining research skills. *Journal of the American Dietetic Association* 2000;100(10):1144–1148.

50. Urden LD. Outcome evaluation: An essential component for CNS practice. *Clinical Nurse Specialist* 1999;13(1):39–46.

51. Reader D, Splett P, Gunderson E. Impact of gestational diabetes mellitus nutrition practice guidelines implemented by registered dietitians on pregnancy outcomes. *Journal of the American Dietetic Association* 2006;106(9):1426–1433.

52. Kuehneman T, Saulsbury D, Splett P, Chapman DB. Demonstrating the impact of nutrition intervention in a heart failure program. *Journal of the American Dietetic Association* 2002;102(12):1790–1794.

53. Splett P, Roth-Yousey L, Vogelzang J. Medical nutrition therapy for the prevention and treatment of unintentional weight loss in residential healthcare facilities. *Journal of the American Dietetic Association* 2003;103(3):352–362.

CHAPTER **8**

The Advanced Practice Approach

"Art is born of the observation and investigation of nature." —*Cicero[1]*

Dietetics is based in science. Indeed, dietitians are widely recognized for having a strong scientific background that supports clinical practice. The previous chapters have described the rigorous education and training proposed for an advanced practice dietitian. With the approach to practice, however, the advanced practice dietitian finds it necessary to switch from the science of MNT to the art of MNT. While the previous sub-themes of the advanced practice model can be supported with literature, the approach to practice is much more abstract. This chapter describes how the advanced practice dietitian refines and applies expertise in the clinical setting. Future research will be needed to provide the scientific detail that supports the advanced practice approach.

The verb "approach" has been defined as "to make advances especially in order to create a desired result."[2] Thus the *approach* used by the advanced practice dietitian entails the application of the knowledge and skills of advanced MNT so as to create a desired result in practice. The advanced practice approach was well defined by participants in the study conducted by this book's authors as comprehensive, discerning, integrated, and simplified. For the purposes of this discussion, "approach" will refer to the application of knowledge and skills in direct patient care, in the practice of MNT, and in the professional work environment.

COMPREHENSIVE APPROACH

"Of course, our failures are a consequence of many factors, but possibly one of the most important is the fact that society operates on the theory that specialization is the key to success, not realizing that specialization precludes comprehensive thinking." —*R. Buckminster Fuller[1]*

The word *comprehensive* has been defined as "covering completely or broadly."[2] It is further defined as "inclusive, as having or exhibiting a wide mental grasp, as in comprehensive knowledge." In previous chapters, advanced practice dietitians demonstrated that they had not only depth, but also breadth of knowledge and skill. They also took a comprehensive view of the patient and the surrounding situation. Thus, for the advanced practice dietitian, the comprehensive approach refers not only to the knowledge of nutrition, but also to the knowledge of the patient, his or her circumstances, and the disease process affecting the patient.

One interviewee mentioned approaching patient information in terms of what was to be done with it, even while considering the theoretical background underlying the patient information. The comprehensive aspect of the approach to practice was described by another dietitian as using her senses in addition to straightforward examination to evaluate a patient. For another, it was expressed as being skilled in "picking up things that others might not have taken time to identify" or "seeing things that a basic level dietitian just doesn't see." Yet another dietitian stated, "And it seems like . . . the depth of your knowledge increases—the depth and breadth of your knowledge and your ability to analyze the entire person versus just parts of the person. And that's where it seems like some of the distinguishing factors [between basic and advanced practice] happen."

The advanced practice dietitians in our study stressed the need to be aware of dynamic or changing situations. As one put it succinctly:

> As dietitians, we have to know the whole picture. And if you miss one of the pieces, then you may have missed a major piece of what is happening to that patient. Without that piece, it could be so far off. As an example, consider an end-of-life issue. Suppose the patient is being extubated so that he or she can die, and you're recommending nutrition support. That is the type of piece that could be missed if you don't take in the whole.

The dietitians in our study had accumulated a great deal of knowledge about patient care and disease process. (This point is illustrated in **Exhibit 8–1.**) Consistent with one of the hallmarks of a true professional, they knew the limitations of their expertise and referred patients to others as needed. More than one dietitian noted that he or she had identified when a patient's symptoms were not related to food and nutrition, but rather derived from some other problem. One dietitian noted that she sometimes identified medical problems in patients referred to her office:

> It's not something that I have the expertise to help them in. But I sure have the ability to pass on the information to the people who do, to get the ball rolling. So I spend a lot of time trying to understand the variables in the person's life. What could be influencing the problems? Whether it's low blood sugar, high blood sugar, weight, or other co-morbidities, I sort of paint the picture in my mind of who that person is with all these things. I send a comprehensive letter to the physician describing all these things. I know that the doctors read them.

Another dietitian had considered the impact of information she obtained from patients:

> Sometimes there are important pieces of information that come out in the nutrition history that impact other parts of treatment. I once provided diet history

EXHIBIT 8–1

Identifying a Co-morbidity in a Patient with Unspecified Dietary Problems

I had a patient come to me once who was referred for dietary problems. I went through everything that she was telling me and I said, "You know, you really need to have a medical workup before we really look at nutritional causes of these problems." To make a long story short, it turned out she had colon cancer. She came back and thanked me. She said if I had just given her a diet, [her doctors] wouldn't have caught [the cancer] as quickly and they wouldn't have been able to do anything about it. She was very, very grateful to me. I just remember thinking to myself that I had argued with the doctor because the doctor was angry at me that I didn't give her a diet. I had felt very strongly that it was inappropriate because she was describing things that could have had medical links—and she did.

When you think "advanced practice," you're thinking outside of the box. You're thinking outside of "How do I have to help this person with his or her diet?" [By "diet,"] I might mean preparation of food, acquiring food, choices of food—anything that has to do with the diet. [Advanced practice requires] thinking outside of that [definition]. Diet is very much a part of everything, but you are aware of everything outside of it as well. It's hard to describe, but it's there.

information that differentiated between liver disease and malnutrition. Another time I identified a family history of hypertriglyceridemia in a patient whose hypertriglyceridemia was attributed to pancreatitis. For a couple of years, I worked with a physician who wouldn't diagnose an eating disorder until I interviewed the patient and discussed the case with him. I didn't make a medical diagnosis in any of these situations, but I did provide information that contributed to the medical diagnosis. It's part of a comprehensive approach.

DISCERNING APPROACH

"The supreme end of education is expert discernment in all things—the power to tell the good from the bad, the genuine from the counterfeit, and to prefer the good and the genuine to the bad and the counterfeit." —Charles Grosvenor Osgood[3]

Discernment has been defined as the ability "to show insight and understanding."[2] In our context, the word "discernment" relates to the ability to individualize activities based on patient need. The advanced practice dietitians in our study used discernment in obtaining and applying information. For example, one interviewee mentioned that she didn't have time to conduct a physical assessment on every patient, but did such assessments "as needed, according to criteria I have in my head."

For another dietitian, discernment was used to easily identify the most important information:

> So now I do a brief look at this baby outside the room, based on what I know I want. I know which questions to ask because I'm looking for specific information. I'm going in to find out the specific information to support or to complete my initial assessment, because I've got 10 minutes with [the child]. I'm not sure you would do that if you didn't have some experience. I have a colleague with whom I've worked for years who hasn't been able to define and hone in on what is important and what is not. She still has to get every detail. She has this fear that she will miss something. In some instances, I would perform like my colleague; in another instance, I would not perform that way, and I guess I'm discerning which place to use it.

In the case mentioned here, the dietitian might be looking for information to confirm the diagnosis. Perhaps she has already talked with the referring physician and is aware of the thinking about the patient. She has probably scanned the medical record, or has heard the medical history during rounds. She may be looking for a few pieces of information to confirm what she has been told, to complete a history, or to shape the intervention she is planning. In any event, the dietitian knows what she needs. She knows which shortcuts she can take and when she can take them.

At the same time, both this dietitian and the one who decides at a glance whether to perform physical assessments have thought in advance about times when more detail is needed. They have discerned their own criteria for obtaining additional information based on extensive practice experience.

Advanced practice dietitians also apply discernment to scientific issues and to the results of the inquiry. For example, they may discard the results of scientific inquiry because it is of poor quality or simply irrelevant. Likewise, they may take a conservative attitude toward new ideas or innovations based on the need for more information or a realization of the complexities of adopting a recommended change in practice. Advanced practice dietitians read the literature and attend conferences, but discern which concepts to apply and discard those that are superfluous. According to one study participant, "They go to a meeting and they put all of that information together, simplify it, bring it back, and apply what they feel is valid.

Some of it's not valid." Another advanced practice dietitian described her sometimes skeptical reaction to new products introduced at a conference by saying, "Just because it's new, it doesn't mean it's the best thing out there. Sometimes it's a marketing issue."

The advanced practice dietitians we studied were discerning in other areas as well. Some had competing priorities such as family and friends, so they were discerning about how to use their time. They were able to limit activities that interfered with family responsibilities and still practice at an advanced level. They avoided wasting time or energy and sought to engage in productive (rather than negative) uses of their time. One described a situation that influenced her discernment of how to use her time:

> You can just waste so much time whining and complaining. Once I worked with a dietitian who spent the first two hours each morning complaining about every aspect of her job and life. It completely sapped the energy of everyone in our office. I learned to avoid the office when she was there. I simply rearranged my day to do office work at a time when she wasn't there. I got so much done that way. The increased productivity elevated my mood. It really taught me to be careful— to use my time positively, not in wasted activity.

INTEGRATED APPROACH

"The whole is greater than the sum of its parts." —*Unknown*

The term *integrated* means to unite with something else or to incorporate into a larger unit. In this case, advanced practice dietitians integrate their assessment, diagnosis, intervention, and monitoring with those of others.[2] Medical care is complex. Not only do patients present with multiple co-morbidities, but they also undergo complex treatments. They have social issues and are subject to family pressures. They experience the stress of economic and job pressures, not to mention the challenges inherent in living in a complex society. An often unrecognized, but preeminent factor in MNT is the social and cultural context surrounding food. To be successful, the advanced practice dietitian must integrate MNT into the patient's life while considering all of these competing factors.

According to participants in our study, the advanced practice dietitian must "help people to understand information and to apply it. Because to me, if we don't apply it at the bedside, it's not worth anything. It's just [a question of] how do you apply it? How do you use it? That's another thing the advanced practitioner does."

One dietitian went so far as to cite the ability to integrate the nutrition intervention into the plan for the patient as defining the difference between basic level and advanced practice dietitians. She stated, "Entry level practice is ['Patients are] malnourished; they need nutrition.' Advanced level practice is 'Yes, but they're dying and they don't want it.'" She went on to say, "That's the difference: recognizing when we should apply medical nutrition therapy and when we should not. It's understanding the appropriateness of application. You have to have a clear understanding of what is the big picture for the patient."

According to another advanced practice dietitian:

> The advanced practice dietitian looks at more than just the nutrition assessment and the proper nutrient prescription. You have to look at what impacts the plan.
>
> There are social factors. Does the patient have resources that will help [him or her] implement what you want [the patient] to do? Will family and friends help? [Does the patient] have social support, economic resources to buy the special foods and products? I worked with a homeless population once. It really makes you think about what you can and can't accomplish.
>
> What about the rest of the treatment plan? What are the medications? How long will the patient be on them? [Is the patient] really diabetic, or [does he or she] just need blood sugar control until the steroids are tapered? These things make a huge difference to patients. They make a huge difference in what you tell them.
>
> Do you know how the physicians who refers [patients] to you typically manage these patients? An advanced practice dietitian asks questions and accumulates this knowledge. An advanced practice dietitian knows the typical course and treatment for diseases within the area of practice. The advanced practice dietitian is able to find out, to communicate with the others involved in care. The advanced practice dietitian knows when various others will be consulted and knows what information to provide so that the nutrition agenda for the patient moves forward.

Advanced practitioners also integrate information, and describe thinking in terms of those relationships and patterns that will enable them to streamline activities, thereby increasing their productivity and effectiveness. Perhaps not surprisingly, the need to integrate therapy within the overall treatment plan was frequently mentioned by study participants. Consider the following example:

> An advanced practitioner RD in diabetes is looking at overall clinical management—not just the MNT piece. Also, you're looking at integrated therapy, and integrating therapy, [which] I would define as the MNT piece, physical activity, and having the strong knowledge base of oral diabetes medication, the various insulin regimens, and the types of insulin. [Advanced practice requires] understanding how that all works together with the diabetes management, and paying attention not just to glucose control but also to blood pressure and lipids.

Interviewees understood the whole treatment plan, knowing when nutrition was a primary concern and when other issues took precedence. These dietitians were very comfortable participating as full-fledged, valued members of the medical team, exhibiting a sense of entitlement regarding their ability to provide nutrition and associated care.

SIMPLIFIED APPROACH

"Everything should be made as simple as possible, but not one bit simpler."
—Albert Einstein[1]

The word *simplified* has been defined as having been reduced to "basic essentials."[2] This word appeared in the vocabulary of advanced practice dietitians when they began discussing how they interacted with complex facts. They were aware that they did not have unlimited time and resources, so they had developed ways to condense or distill information to its most essential elements while still achieving the best results.

One advanced MNT practitioner described thinking in terms of relationships and patterns that enabled the dietitian to streamline activities, targeting key issues as appropriate. For another, it was an issue of simplicity:

The advanced practitioner makes it look simple. . . . goes in and looks at all that's around to come up with a summation. And it looks simple to the outsider, but that's where the novice doesn't realize the training and all the background that it took to get to that point—to synthesize complex information and to make it simplified in order to apply it to clinical practice.

Other practitioners used a simplified approach based on extensive experience. They developed hierarchies of information that was needed or even useful. They isolated the single, simplest, most effective intervention that would achieve the desired results, or they attacked the simplest explanations first (see **Exhibit 8–2** for an example). The advanced practice dietitians were able to see which intervention would improve the situation and target the questions in the history toward that line of thinking.

SUMMARY

This chapter used the words of advanced practice dietitians to describe the approach they use in applying their expertise to nutrition care of patients. This ap-

EXHIBIT 8-2

Getting to the Simplest Issue First

When you work in critical care, the data at your fingertips are so seductive. You find more and more information about the patient each day on rounds. If you're not very careful, you can develop what businesspeople call "paralysis of analysis." Instead of thinking about the cause of the problem, you call for more data, more information, or more treatment.

If the patient on a tube feeding develops diarrhea, the basic level dietitians will start ordering labs, manipulating or changing the formula, asking for medications. There's this big flurry of activity.

In fact, 9 times out of 10, a quick review of the medication record and flow sheets will tell the tale. You really can't accomplish anything until you find out what else is going down that tube. More often than not, the patient was given potassium chloride or some other electrolytes. [Or perhaps] a cathartic was ordered because the patient hadn't had a bowel movement in several days. There is a temporal relationship. It's rarely the feeding that is the root of the problem, but it takes experience to be able to identify [the real problem] and lots of confidence not to react with lots of unnecessary activity.

proach is difficult to describe and even more difficult to measure. Nevertheless, these descriptions should increase understanding of how advanced MNT is practiced.

KEY POINTS

- The advanced practice dietitian in MNT obtains comprehensive information about the patient and his or her concurrent treatment plan.
- The advanced practice dietitian discerns which information is valuable in a particular situation and acts on it. He or she identifies information that is important to others and communicates it appropriately. The advanced practice dietitian also discerns information that is superfluous or of poor quality, and discards or does not act on that information.

- The advanced practice dietitian integrates nutrition therapy into the larger plan of care, adjusting the MNT as needed in the face of complex and dynamic situations.
- The advanced practice dietitian targets MNT to obtain the best possible results.

SUGGESTED READING

Groopman J. *How doctors think*. New York: Houghton-Mifflin, 2007.

This readable book, which is designed for the layperson, details how doctors diagnose disease and how errors in medical judgment occur.

Montgomery K. *How doctors think*. London: Oxford Press, 2006.

This book provides an academic perspective on the application of scientific knowledge to the practice of medicine.

EXPERIENCES TO TRY

1. Go to Wikipedia and read about Occam's razor. Can you apply this thinking to your practice?

2. Think of a patient you have seen within the last two or three days. As you think of your approach to that patient, ask yourself the following questions:

   - Have I been comprehensive? Do I have all the information about this situation that I need? Is there any value in obtaining more information from the patient or the family? Is there any value in obtaining more information from other health professionals?

   - Have I been discerning? What is the quality of information I have? If I had more information, how would it affect my intervention? Where am I making assumptions based on hearsay rather than checking out matters for myself? Where am I relying on textbooks rather than current literature? Is there extraneous information that I can discard? Is there anything that I need to discuss with others to broaden my perspective?

   - Have I integrated my plan into the priorities for the patient? What was the highest medical priority for the patient today? Will this priority change between now and the next time I see the patient? How does the nutrition intervention further the overall treatment plan for this patient? Have I discussed my plan with the attending physician? With the nurses caring for the patient?

- Have I used the simplest approach? Will the intervention I've selected correct the most important nutrition problem or improve the etiology of the nutrition diagnosis?

(Repeat this exercise every few days until you are comfortable that you are using an advanced practice approach.)

REFERENCES

1. The quotations page. Available at http://www.quotationspage.com/subjects/. Accessed May 19, 2007.
2. Merriam-Webster Online. Available at www.m-w.com/. Accessed July 5, 2006.
3. Apocrypha. The Samuel Johnson sound bite page. Available at http://www.samuel johnson.com/apocryph.html#2. Accessed June 3, 2007.

Influencing Patients, Practice, and the Environment

"Setting an example is not the main means of influencing another; it is the only means." —Albert Einstein[1]

The previous chapters in this text described in global terms the knowledge and skills that advanced practice dietitians state are characteristic of their practice. These descriptions highlighted the necessary education, experience, and credentials that support advanced practice. They provided insight into the practice context and the attitude of the advanced practice dietitian. Advanced practice dietitians also described their expertise and their approach to practice.

The current chapter describes how the components of the advanced practice model are applied in the work environment. It offers numerous examples of how the advanced practice dietitian affects individual patients, practice, and the larger environment in which MNT is delivered.

PATIENTS

"To know and not to do is not to know." —Unknown

A *patient* is "an individual under medical care and treatment," whereas a *client* is "a person who engages the professional advice or services of another."[2] The advanced practice dietitian providing MNT works directly with patients and clients using modifications in food and nutrient intake to improve health or prevent disease. The primary role of the advanced practice dietitian in MNT is direct patient care. Although he or she often has other important roles, these duties remain secondary to providing MNT directly to patients or clients.

The advanced practice dietitian may see patients with a specific medical diagnosis, such as diabetes or renal disease. He or she may also see patients receiving a certain type of therapy, such as enteral nutrition or counseling for weight reduction. Furthermore, the advanced practice dietitian may work in a specific setting, such as in a neonatal intensive care unit or in home care. Nevertheless, the delivery of care to a patient population with a specific medical diagnosis, requiring a specific type of therapy, or in a particular location does little to distinguish the basic from the advanced level of practice. Instead of focusing on the type of patient, it seems more consistent to define advanced practice based on the activities of the dietitian.

At least three characteristics of the advanced practice dietitian's interaction with the patients will likely serve to define the advanced practice dietitian's impact on patients:

- *Autonomy.* The advanced practice dietitian must have the confidence to function autonomously within the practice setting.
- *Expert intervention.* The advanced practice dietitian must provide interventions to achieve results that document the value of the dietetics services.
- *Treatment of complex nutritional problems.* The advanced practice dietitian must be able to effectively manage complex problems to demonstrate value.

Thus the advanced practice dietitian functions autonomously, as a consultant providing expert intervention to patients or clients with complex nutrition-related diagnoses.

Autonomy

The first of the three unique factors distinguishing advanced practice is autonomy. The advanced practice dietitian has the confidence to function without direct supervision, but collaboratively with others. Such a professional is confident enough to do more than just "recommend"; that is, the advanced practice dietitian "does" rather than "knows." Advanced practice dietitians fulfill a professional role, taking calls, participating in a practice that requires seven-days-per-week coverage, and adjusting their hours to meet the needs of clients or referring physicians. In short, they accept responsibility for patients outside normal working hours.

Advanced practice dietitians are also autonomous in initiating interventions. They typically have clinical privileges to order diets, enteral feedings, or parenteral feedings; perform tests and procedures; refer patients for consultation; and manipulate medications. **Exhibit 9–1** examines the levels of autonomy applied to manipulation of phosphate binders. In dialysis centers, advanced practice dietitians may have clinical privileges to order diets, and some may manipulate other nutrition-related medications. The same model is used in acute care hospitals, where dietitians may be privileged to write parenteral nutrition orders or independently order lab tests for the purpose of monitoring therapy.[3,4] In outpatient clinics, dietitians determine the appropriate diets for patients and order laboratory tests as necessary to monitor their interventions.[5] This model also extends to long-term care and rehabilitation facilities.[6,7]

Expert Intervention

Throughout the text, exhibits have described the level of expertise that advanced practice dietitians bring to the interventions that they provide. In the course of our research, we have seen dietitians who instantly shift from one intervention to

EXHIBIT 9-1

Levels of Autonomy in a Dialysis Clinic

The patient presents in clinic with an elevated serum phosphorus level. The dietitian takes a history from the patient and determines that there has been no change in the phosphorus intake from usual. The dietitian inquires as to whether the patient is taking the phosphate binders as prescribed. The patient is taking the phosphate binders, a fact verified by a family member. The dietitian may address the need for a change in the dose of phosphate binders in one of three ways.

Basic Level Practice. The dietitian practicing at the basic level notes the findings in the medical record and recommends to the physician that the phosphate binders be increased.

Practice by Preapproved Protocol. The dialysis center may have a preapproved protocol in place, outlining the means by which the dietitian can adjust the phosphorus binders according to the serum phosphorus levels. For example, the dialysis center may have a preapproved protocol that states the dietitian can increase the dose of lanthanum carbonate from 750 to 1000 mg if the patient has a phosphorus level between 5.0 and 5.5 mg/dL, and increase the dose of lanthanum carbonate to 1500 mg if the phosphorus level is between 5.6 and 6.0 mg/dL.*

Practice by Clinical Privileges. The dietitian has presented credentials to the medical staff who oversee credentialing for the dialysis center. In this center, the dietitian has clinical privileges to independently (without physician co-signature) manipulate food and nutrient intake and phosphate binders so as to keep the patient's serum phosphorus levels within a predetermined range. He or she must demonstrate ongoing continuing education to maintain these clinical privileges, which are granted for a finite period of time.

* This information is provided as an illustration of a clinical protocol. It is not a recommendation for patient management. All health professionals are required to review the appropriate prescribing information prior to recommending or ordering any drug.

another as the patient's course of treatment changes. We have encountered dietitians who were able to identify problems that others had missed. We have witnessed the depth of counseling skills provided by advanced practice dietitians. Clearly, the advanced practice dietitian possesses in-depth knowledge of MNT. In addition, he or she is extraordinarily skillful in using that expertise to craft effective nutritional interventions. Thus the advanced practice dietitian not only "knows," but also "does."

Treatment of Complex Nutritional Problems

The third component of the advanced practice dietitian's practice is the complex patient. *Complexity* may be defined as "hard to separate, analyze, or solve."[2] Thus a complex patient could be one whose nutrition diagnosis was difficult to identify. The advanced practice dietitian would have the skill to unravel the most complex nutrition diagnoses and treat them with the simplest or most complex interventions. By focusing on the nutrition diagnosis and the nutrition intervention, rather than on the medical diagnosis, it becomes easier to identify the contributions made by the advanced practice dietitian. This approach also aids in answering the inevitable question—"So what does an advanced practice dietitian do that a regular dietitian does not?"—that is asked when advanced practice dietitians request additional compensation based on their increased level of responsibility (see **Table 9–1**).

Additional Patient-Related Roles

Advanced practice dietitians typically function as consultants. They generally do not see patients automatically according to policy, as the result of screening, or because they are admitted to a certain location of a healthcare institution. Rather, the advanced practice dietitian is consulted by another health professional—usually a physician—and asked to contribute his or her nutritional expertise to patient management. The fact that advanced practice dietitians must be consulted to see a patient increases the value of their interventions in the minds of both patient and referring caregiver. It also places these dietitians on a par with other consultants, including physicians, advanced practice nurses, social workers, and physical therapists. In the hospital or other institution, advanced practice dietitians are consulted by physicians, physician assistants, or nurse practitioners. In the community or in private practice, they maintain referral networks consisting of the same professionals. Also, in the community, advanced practice dietitians may accept self-referred patients.

Table 9-1 Distinguishing Between Basic and Advanced Levels of Practice

	Basic Level of Practice	Advanced Level of Practice
Source of patients	The basic level dietitian sees patients according to his or her location within an institution or as the result of screening.	The advanced practice dietitian sees patients who are referred by a physician or other provider. The dietitian recognizes these referral sources and nurtures these relationships. A consult is required to allow order writing or for billing purposes.
Patient relationship	Episodic; a single encounter or a single encounter with a single follow-up. The nature and details of the encounter are specified by policy (e.g., patients on certain types of diets are seen for education; patients are seen because of a certain length of stay).	Ongoing; the patient is seen daily, weekly, or at another regular interval. The dietitian exercises autonomy in working with the patient to determine the duration of the intervention (e.g., patients are seen until the nutrition diagnosis is stable or resolved; then the dietitian signs off the case, or the dietitian and patient agree to stop therapy).
Primary patient care activities	Nutrition assessment, nutrition education.	Nutrition diagnosis, nutrition intervention, monitoring nutrition outcomes.
Administrative activities	Occasionally attends meetings; participates in activities as directed by a supervisor or manager.	Selects which meetings to attend; participates in activities according to available time and practice priorities. Manages time to accommodate a variety of roles, including teaching, clinical research, marketing, and self-education.
Role contacts	Patients, other dietitians, nurses, and occasionally physicians. Primary contacts are within the work setting.	Patients, physicians, and sometimes nurses, pharmacists, administrators, and others as needed. Primary contacts are within the work setting, but there are many outside contacts that provide and request information.
Level of autonomy	Makes recommendations based on the patient's medical diagnosis or laboratory data. Rarely knows the outcome of these recommendations.	Independently orders—without a verbal order or physician co-signature—meals, snacks, enteral or parenteral nutrition, and necessary monitoring. Measures outcomes and adjusts interventions.

In addition to providing direct patient care, advanced practice dietitians may have responsibilities in teaching, research, or administration:

- Frequently, advanced practice dietitians serve as preceptors, course directors, or visiting faculty. They may teach dietetics, pharmacy, nursing, or medical students, residents, or fellows. They may have adjunct faculty appointments in medicine, surgery, nursing, or pharmacy as well as in dietetics.

- In some situations, advanced practice dietitians participate in clinical research studies. They may provide support or advice from the nutrition perspective for studies within their work environment. They may conduct their own clinical research projects or collaborate with other clinical researchers.
- Advanced practice dietitians may have administrative responsibilities such as developing and implementing practice guidelines or protocols. They may contribute to their workgroup by finding and organizing practice information.

While they may not fulfill all these roles within their practice, advanced practice dietitians perform multiple roles that demonstrate their intellect and are also a measure of initiative. Several examples of advanced practice roles are found in **Table 9–2.**

Table 9–2 Examples of Advanced Practice Roles

· A credentialed dietitian in diabetes education with years of experience in dialysis works as a joint practitioner with a group of nephrologists and nurses. This dietitian allocates 5% of her time to adjunct faculty appointments in two dietetics programs and has collaborated with a group at the state level to collect outcomes data related to dietetics services for pre-dialysis patients with diabetes.

· A dietitian with years of experience in a neonatal intensive care unit and follow-up clinic has developed a joint practice with a group of obstetricians who refer women for nutrition care during pregnancy. In addition, she follows these women for weight reduction and infant feeding issues after birth. This dietitian also provides education for dietitians in her area of practice through a national continuing education provider.

· An experienced nutrition support dietitian has obtained clinical privileges to order parenteral and enteral nutrition, including related tests, procedures, and medications, according to an established scope of practice. This dietitian is sought after as a speaker and has worked with critical care physicians and nurses to collect and evaluate data reducing sepsis in his units.

· A coordinator of a multiyear clinical trial that involves counseling patients to maintain nutrition behavior change has participated in dozens of clinical trials and industry-funded contracts. This dietitian supervises the activities of clinical trial dietitians at six different sites, but spends 50% of her time in direct patient care and 5% of her time teaching a class for a local university.

· The clinical coordinator for a dietetics program works with students three days per week and manages the nutrition component of a weight-control clinic for a physician group two days per week. The dietitian collects outcomes data on her patients for a project to demonstrate the value of nutrition counseling of obese patients for insurance companies.

PRACTICE

A *practice* may be defined as "the continuous exercise of a profession."[2] As mentioned in Chapter 2, in most professions approximately 10 years of continuous practice is required to perform at the expert level. One of the reasons for this requirement is that the individual must develop sufficient continuous experience to provide a basis for reflective practice. The advanced practice dietitian has enough practice experience to think in terms of a group of patients and to recognize how they react to their disease processes and the accompanying nutritional interventions. Based on his or her extensive experience, the advanced practice dietitian can recognize patterns of signs and symptoms, thereby permitting the correct nutrition diagnosis and selection of the most effective nutritional intervention. The dietitian uses this experience to reflect on the "rules" or "conventional wisdom" supporting the choice of particular nutritional interventions for certain groups of patients, and then questions why things are done in a certain way for these patients. Careful reflection at this level leads to experimentation with new nutritional interventions, subsequent testing of those interventions, and, eventually, improvements in practice.

The advanced practice dietitian is able to anticipate the response to nutritional interventions based on experience, knowing both what is typical for the situation and how to modify interventions successfully for the atypical situation. The advanced practice dietitian may make comments such as "We usually see stomatitis on day 3 with this type of chemotherapy, and we work with the patients to modify diet texture until symptoms resolve about two weeks later. Not all of our patients develop stomatitis, however, so we don't modify the diet unless it's needed."

The advanced practice dietitian typically keeps patient records, but he or she may also maintain a patient registry or database in an effort to identify issues with nutritional intervention and to track changes in interventions. Reviewing these records or querying the database then enables the dietitian to identify problematic issues with certain interventions. As a result, the advanced practice dietitian begins to speak in terms of incidence or prevalence of nutrition-related issues in a given patient population.

For example, one advanced practice dietitian cited the following evolution of knowledge about a nutrition-related problem:

> [Approximately] 25% of our patients experience refeeding hypophosphatemia despite receiving no more than 25 kilocalories per kilogram of body weight. We've learned that the risk factors in the literature don't really help us to identify the [patients whose phosphorus levels drop]. We're looking at a protocol to

help with that. We really don't worry too much about potassium with refeeding because we looked at 250 of our patients and really didn't see anyone with a big drop within the first four days of feeding.

At some point, advanced practice dietitians may accumulate enough experience with specific groups of patients to publish their observations of a series of patients, or they may identify questions that should be answered to improve the nutritional interventions used in a certain patient population. They may publish outcome studies based on their findings. Some dietitians may advance practice by designing and testing new interventions. They may also identify and discard ineffective interventions, thereby reducing resource utilization rates or streamlining care. All of these activities share a common foundation: the use of data to improve patient care.

Over time, the advanced practice dietitian spends enough time reflecting on practice issues and discussing these issues with colleagues to develop a clearly articulated practice philosophy. This philosophy may encompass issues related to patients, provide a framework for dealing with recurring but complicated issues, or provide a framework for approaching new information or unfamiliar situations. Such a practice philosophy will typically acknowledge the place of nutritional interventions in patient care; elucidate relationships with patients, other professionals, students, and support staff; and perhaps lay out practitioner biases. An excerpt from one advanced practice dietitian's practice philosophy appears in **Exhibit 9–2.**

EXHIBIT 9–2

An Advanced Practice Dietitian's Practice Philosophy

Because of some of my early experiences while diabetes care was developing, I have a conservative practice philosophy. Because I've watched practice develop, I believe that we can never stop learning, and never stop challenging what we know. However, I've seen lots of new interventions that were discarded because they harmed patients, even if harm was only defined as a waste of money. I believe in innovation, but I also believe in measuring or tracking the results of what we do. Sometimes it's surprising how real patient data differ from perceptions. That's because we tend to remember the single outstanding case rather than the 30 routine ones. Data help us form more objective opinions about the interventions we provide and how well they work.

continues

EXHIBIT 9–2 *continued*

> We have an obligation to use resources wisely based on what will work, not just based on what is new. We owe it to our patients to carefully consider the simplest and most streamlined approach that will be effective for them. In each case, we have to look at the total patient. Can our patients (or the team caring for them) manage the therapy we provide? How will it improve their quality of life? Is it worth it to them? Our patients can teach us a great deal if we take the time to follow them closely and to find out how they react. We have to keep up with what's new in the literature, but also create that literature based on what we learn by observing the patients in our practice.

ENVIRONMENT

The *environment* may be defined as "the circumstances, objects, or conditions by which one is surrounded."[2] The practice environment differs from the "environment of care" that is a part of institutional accreditation,[8] instead referring to the influences on patients and practice. The advanced practice dietitian is not only aware of and influenced by the environment, but also influences that environment.

Environment begins with the "corporate culture" of the institution, which may be formally described in documents such as mission, vision, and values statements. Corporate or organizational culture also includes unstated dimensions, such as the formality, respect, and distance within staff and between staff and patients and the work style of the employees at all levels. This culture is inevitably influenced by the institutional sponsorship—that is, whether the organization at hand is a religious order, community, government, educational institution, or for-profit organization. In addition, corporate culture shapes work or performance standards, the level of practice, the focus on fiscal responsibility, and academic rigor.

Likewise, the practice environment is shaped by the neighborhood where the dietitian practices—whether it is rural or urban, affluent or poor. In addition, the ethnicity and cultural background of the patients and the staff affect the environment. The environment may differ depending on the institution's location, including the distance to competing facilities and transportation issues that arise because of its location. Finally, the practice environment may be heavily influenced by the case mix of the patients served, the number who have private insurance, the number who are indigent, and the institutional mission (e.g., caring for women, children, veterans, or retired members of a certain organization).

An even larger environment is the one circumscribed by regulations. In most states, dietetic practice is regulated by licensure laws that specify what dietitians do. Other regulations at the municipality, county, state, and federal levels may also affect dietitians, given that they are designed to regulate practice. Such rules are interpreted differently in different settings, which accounts for the variability in practice by setting and by institution. The details of these regulations and their interpretation are beyond the scope of this book; a key to locating them appears in **Table 9–3.**

Table 9–3 Examples of Organizations That Influence the Environment of Dietetics Practice

Federal Level

U.S. Department of Agriculture
Department of Health and Human Services
Centers for Medicare and Medicaid Services
National Institutes of Health
Centers for Disease Control and Prevention
Food and Drug Administration
National Academy of Science
Agency for Healthcare Research and Quality

State Level

State Departments of Health
State Licensure Boards
State Business and Professional Code
State Facility Licensing Bodies

Professional Organizations

American Dietetic Association
Commission on Accreditation of Dietetic Education
Commission on Dietetic Registration
American Heart Association
American Diabetes Association
Society of Critical Care Medicine
American Society for Parenteral and Enteral Nutrition
Council on Renal Nutrition

Private Organizations

Leapfrog Group
Joint Commission
Healthcare Facilities Accreditation Program

Another environment comprises the professional organizations that provide resources for dietitians. Many of these organizations depend on the expertise of advanced practice dietitians to develop standards, guidelines, or protocols for practice, education, or credentialing.

Ultimately, however, the advanced practice dietitian envisions the environment as being even larger. That is, he or she will be aware of the level of practice within a state or national group, will talk about issues at the level of the profession, and understands the political influences on practice issues such as licensure and reimbursement. In our study, advanced practice dietitians indicated that their environment was large, extending to the level of the profession and beyond to the regulatory environment.

A differentiating factor between basic and advanced level practice is the perceived ability to influence the practice environment. The basic level practitioner gradually becomes aware of the practice environment and slowly begins to react to it. By contrast, the advanced practice dietitian actively moves to influence or shape the environment, rather than simply reacting to it. Such a dietitian exhibits a proactive stance, anticipating changes in the environment and developing ways to influence those changes. The advanced practice dietitian may obtain and present information substantiating a needed change; indeed, he or she is highly skilled in gathering and using data to drive change. Clearly, the advanced practice dietitian understands the entities that influence practice and uses a finely tuned sense of timing to advance the practice agenda.

Not surprisingly, the advanced practice dietitian is familiar with organizational structures, rules, and laws. From personal experience, he or she understands how guidelines and policies are developed. As part of his or her proactive stance, such a dietitian takes advantage of informed sources to aid in interpreting licensure laws, practice acts, regulations, and standards. In addition, the advanced practice dietitian works to strengthen professional organizations and enhance their influence over the policies that govern practice.

According to participants in our study, a defining characteristic of the advanced practice dietitian is his or her willingness to make contributions to the field. This may be done through formal communication, such as writing papers or presenting at conferences. It may also occur informally, by influencing leaders in professional, regulatory, or governmental organizations. As one advanced practice dietitian stated:

> You may need to publish or speak, or influence legislation or policy. It may be a
> national effort or just [a discussion] within a circle of colleagues. You may teach,
> but you get your ideas and experience out there. They may benefit others, who
> can learn from your expertise. [Such activity] also meets a need to test yourself,

to test your expertise, to see if what you know stands up in a larger arena. It's a way of validating your thinking. It's not about recognition; it's about finding a group of like-minded individuals who collaborate to move an agenda forward. This group may be in your village or city, or it may be international.

The vehicle for communication isn't the important thing: It's the level of the conversation. It's the level of the intellectual or clinical challenge. Is that why one participates in academia, or consults in extremely difficult cases that others could not solve, or works in a difficult or demanding area of practice, or testifies in court as an expert witness, or writes articles, or convinces a huge organization to move in a different direction? I think that's it. It's a way of testing one's initiative and skill.

There are people who are very vocal [in insisting] that writing and speaking should not be a part of the criteria for advanced practice, and they may be right. However, recognition has been correlated with advanced practice in at least one model. I'm not saying that recognition is a prerequisite for advanced practice; it's not. Recognition is probably the result.

SUMMARY

The advanced practice dietitian in MNT formulates the advanced practice attitude, aptitude, context, and expertise into an approach to patients, practice, and the practice environment. His or her primary role is to serve as a consultant, autonomously providing expert nutritional interventions to patients or clients who have complex nutrition diagnoses. In addition, the advanced practice dietitian reflects on practice and develops an approach to a group of patients that is continually adjusted based on changing information, which is gathered by studying patients' responses to interventions or by keeping up-to-date on new scientific findings. The advanced practice dietitian interacts with the environment at the practice setting, profession, and governmental levels to test ideas, share information, and influence practice, the profession, the healthcare environment, and those state and national organizations that drive nutritional policies.

KEY POINTS

- The advanced practice dietitian not only "knows," but also "does." He or she is distinguished not only by the ability to provide expert interventions, but also by the autonomy that allows the dietitian to practice independently.
- The advanced practice dietitian reflects on his or her experience with a group of patients, and then evaluates practice in an effort to improve interventions.

- The advanced practice dietitian uses data within and outside the work setting to improve practice.
- The advanced practice dietitian actively interacts with the practice environment and shapes that environment.

SUGGESTED READING

Hager M. Hospital therapeutic diet orders and the Centers for Medicare and Medicaid Services: Steering through regulations to provide quality nutrition care and avoid survey citations. *Journal of the American Dietetic Association* 2006;106:198–204.

Hager M, Otto M. To cosign or not to cosign: What managers need to consider. *Journal of the American Dietetic Association* 2006;106:1328–1332.

Hager M, Otto M. An introduction to government regulations and the profession of dietetics. *Journal of the American Dietetic Association* 2006;106:1156–1159.

Handy CB. *Understanding organizations,* 3rd ed. New York, NY. Harmondsworth: Penguin Books, 1985.

This classic management text explains organizational or corporate culture.

Herzlinger RE. *Consumer-driven health care: Implications for providers, payers, and policy-makers.* San Francisco, CA: Jossey-Bass, 2004.

A noted Harvard professor provides thoughts on the healthcare environment.

How to use and understand statutes, regulations, guidelines, interpretations and model guidance. Chicago: American Society for Healthcare Risk Management, 2003. Available at www.ASHRM.org. Accessed May 18, 2007.

This publication is designed for risk managers, but is a brief and useful guide to understanding the origin of the "rules" by which we practice.

Silver H, Moreland K, Skipper A. *The ADA guide to obtaining clinical privileges and nutrition order writing.* Chicago: American Dietetic Association, 2008.

EXPERIENCES TO TRY

1. Locate and read a copy of the licensure law for your state; it should be available on the website of your state government. Locate and read a copy of the Scope of Dietetics Practice and Framework on the American Dietetic Association's website or in *Journal of the American Dietetic Association* and, if one has been developed, a copy of Standards of Professional Performance for your area of practice. Using the examples in the Scope Dietetics Practice and Framework, what support do you observe for an advanced practice role? Do you see the possibility to legislate a change in the licensure law in your state to increase the opportunities for advanced practice dietitians? How have nurse practitioners approached this issue in your state?

2. Attend Public Policy Week in Washington, D.C. This meeting, which is held each spring, offers an opportunity for dietitians to understand and influence policy at the federal level. Similar activities usually occur annually in each state.

3. Go to the Internet and use a search engine to search on the term "locus of control." Many instruments are available that test for locus of control. Locate one such instrument and complete it, and then read about locus of control. How does your individual score on this instrument influence your thinking about your ability to influence your work environment?

REFERENCES

1. Wisdom quotes. Available at http://www.wisdomquotes.com/002629.html. Accessed April 17, 2007.
2. Merriam-Webster Online. Available at www.m-w.com/. Accessed July 5, 2006.
3. Mueller C. Advanced practice in clinical dietetics: Clinical privileges. *Support Line* 2005;27(6):3–5.
4. Rogers D, Fish JA. Entry-level dietetics practice today: Results from the 2005 Commission on Dietetic Registration entry-level dietetics practice audit. *Journal of the American Dietetic Association* 2006;106(6):957–964.e922.
5. Myers EF, Barnhill G, Bryk J. Clinical privileges: Missing piece of the puzzle for clinical standards that elevate responsibilities and salaries for registered dietitians. *Journal of the American Dietetic Association* 2002;102(1):123–132.
6. Wildish DE. Medical directive: Authorizing dietitians to write diet and tube-feeding orders. *Canadian Journal of Dietetic Practice and Research* 2001;62(4):204–206.
7. Moreland K, Gotfried M, Vaughn L. Development and implementation of the clinical privileges for dietitian nutrition order writing program at a long-term acute-care hospital. *Journal of the American Dietetic Association* 2002;102(1):72–74.
8. *2006 Comprehensive Accreditation Manual for Hospitals: The Official Handbook.* Oakbrook, IL: Joint Commission, 2006.

Application of the Advanced Practice Model

"If we are to survive, we must have ideas, vision, and courage. These things are rarely produced by committees. Everything that matters in our intellectual and moral life begins with an individual confronting his own mind and conscience in a room by himself." —*Arthur M. Schlesinger, Jr.* [1]

PUTTING THE ADVANCED PRACTICE MODEL TO WORK

Dietitians who desire to assume an advanced practice role must obtain the knowledge and skills required to perform at the advanced practice level, but may also need information about how to implement that role. This chapter contains a collection of information that may serve as examples for those wishing to implement an advanced practice role. It also includes two interviews with advanced practice dietitians: one who works in a transplant section in a major medical center (**Exhibit**

10–1) and one who maintains a private practice in nutrition and genetics and also writes and teaches nutrition in genetics (**Exhibit 10–2**). These examples are typical of the advanced practice role, but dozens of others exist in all facets of MNT.

The remainder of this chapter presents examples of some of the protocols and policies needed to implement an advanced practice role. In some settings, advanced practice dietitians work without formalizing their roles. This practice is changing, however, as licensure, regulations, and scope of practice issues emerge. For dietitians in an institutional setting, the example of a career ladder incorporating advanced practice may prove useful (**Table 10–1**). A sample application for clinical privileges is presented in **Table 10–2**. The policy related to clinical privileges (**Table 10–3**) may also prove useful for those working in a medical center. The sample collaborative practice agreement in **Table 10–4** may serve as a guide for an advanced practice dietitian working in a clinic, diabetes center, or dialysis clinic.

EXHIBIT 10–1

An Interview with Laura Matarese, Ph.D., R.D., FADA, CNSD (an Advanced Practice Dietitian Working in Intestinal Transplantation)*

What are the types of things that you do?

I divide my job into the areas of research, administration, patient care, patient education, and professional education. It seems as if I do a little of each of these every day. For professional education, it may involve lecturing at a conference or development of an educational program; other times I'm with students on site. We also have classes for our patients.

I'm very independent with patient care. I had to learn the transplant piece and post-transplant part of things. I see the patients as they are being evaluated or listed for transplantation. If they have difficulty eating after transplantation, I assist them in the transition. For those who are PN [parenteral

*Dr. Matarese's official title is Director of Nutrition, Intestinal Rehabilitation and Transplantation Center, Thomas E. Starzl Transplantation Institute, University of Pittsburgh Medical Center.

EXHIBIT 10–1 *continued*

nutrition] dependent, I write their orders. We have some patients who are at home on PN and are stable. Then they come in and do really well post-transplant. I work with them on their appetite and adjust their micronutrients. Many of them need vitamins or trace elements.

For the research side of things, I'm expected to present at conferences, write up the results of the things we do here. Of course, I'm the PI [primary investigator] on my dissertation study, and I'm on several NIH-funded projects as a consultant. Then I do prospective research with our patients. Currently, I am investigating the micronutrient requirements of patients following small bowel and multivisceral transplantation. My dissertation research was presented at an international meeting. I put together an abstract based on some preliminary data. I also observed that a small cohort of our population became obese, and so I reported on that. Where we are in the march of science, it's still possible to present descriptive or observational data. We have also done some prospective research on the quality of life following intestinal transplantation.

The administrative part of my job includes the development of a database for the PN patients. We also wrote a patient education manual, which was much needed. I spend some time writing letters to insurance companies to get approval for PN—the insurance companies need just the right documentation.

Another thing I've done since I've been here is brainstorming with the other sections outside transplant that may not think of nutrition. We have people who are doing basic research, and I've introduced the concept of getting people to communicate and establish an Institute of Nutrition. One of the things related to that is the proposal I put together for a nutrition support handbook.

I think the future for dietitians is bright if they get advanced training. This will also go a long way toward improving the image of dietitians. There are a lot of dietitians who let their job drive their practice, rather than their

continues

EXHIBIT 10–1 *continued*

practice driving their job. For example, here the dietitians began writing the PN. It happened when the chief of the medical staff said, "I think it's time for the dietitians to write the PN." He initiated it. Of course, they had to have a CNSD. Of course, with privilege comes responsibility; some will embrace this, whereas others will not. We need to attract innovative and forward-thinking individuals who can see new things and make them happen. This also requires knowledge and new skill sets. Of course, we need the ambition to conceptualize and make things happen.

One advantage of my job is that I work for the transplant service, so I have a lot of freedom to do things, to make changes. When I took this job, I didn't have a job description. I had a letter with three bullet points outlining my general responsibilities. I'm still creating as I go. This was a new job, a new institution, and new patients, so I was really able to be creative.

I have a lot of independence. The patients are complex, and I am fortunate to be part of a multidisciplinary team. The days here are never boring. They aren't very routine. When I do patient care, I'm mostly on the outpatient side. I have three clinic days—but that's growing, so the other days I write and do administrative work. Most advanced practice dietitians write. Also, I like doing new things. I am always happiest breaking new ground.

One of the nice things about this job is the faculty appointment. That's something that I asked for during the interview process. This was primarily philosophical for me. However, there are some benefits that come along with it: travel funds, funds for dues, parking, and a cell phone. Of course, with my Ph.D., I'm eligible to become Assistant Professor.

As far as my advice for dietitians wishing to move into an advanced practice role, it would be to learn as much as you can. Try to think creatively. Think of a concept, and then plan for it. True success comes from hard work. Of course, you have to sustain that work; you have to keep producing. You have to have the skills and do the work. That's the way to command a decent salary.

EXHIBIT 10–2

An Interview with Ruth DeBusk, Ph.D., RD (an Advanced Practice Dietitian Working in Nutrition and Genetics)

How does nutritional genomics relate to clinical practice?

There are two approaches.

First, because of their slightly different genes, people are phenotypically different. It's these genetic variations that affect how well individuals metabolize a particular nutrient or break down their food, how much they absorb—all the individual variations make them phenotypically unique. There is no such thing as a Dietary Reference Intakes (DRI) for a whole population, because each individual is going to need more or less.

Second, there is a really exciting part from the therapeutic or prevention standpoint. Food has bioactive components within it that act on genes, turning gene expression on or off. So you could be ramping down inflammation or making yourself more heart healthy. You could rev up your detoxification genes. Even though you have a genetic susceptibility for a specific disease, you may not develop [that disease] if you make the appropriate food and lifestyle choices. I see this directly within the purview of the registered dietitian.

What does a genetics practitioner do?

Everything from classical genetics and inborn errors of metabolism to nutritional genomics that focuses on developing nutritional interventions based on the individual's genetic makeup. In the GI area, we do a lot with colon cancer, celiac disease (gluten-sensitive enteropathy), and inflammatory bowel disorders. Ulcerative colitis and Crohn's disease look very similar clinically, but we're beginning to be able to distinguish them genetically. We look at a person's Phase I and Phase II liver detoxification capabilities and then structure nutrition therapy accordingly. The practitioner of the future is going to order and interpret genetic analyses, and then translate this insight into what the client is going to have for dinner.

continues

EXHIBIT 10–2 *continued*

I would love to see something for dietitians like [the credential for] the nurse practitioner role, where there's a fair amount or even total autonomy. The dietitian would own that end of health care. We would have the assertiveness and the confidence to own it, to let everybody know we own it, and to be undisputedly the experts at what we do. If we could get there, we are going to be looking at a unique niche that enables us to increase our therapeutic effectiveness significantly, which will lead to much better income and career satisfaction as well as enhanced respect for the profession. Our patients will tell everybody they know—and then you've got a booming practice.

What is the career path for a nutritional genomics practitioner?

I would start out as a dietitian, but would ideally know where I was going from the very beginning. Don't take what I call "science lite." You need to know how to use the primary literature as your source of information—not some textbook or magazine to document what you're doing. If the physician wants you to talk about the documentation for what you do, you need to have that on the tip of your tongue. As long as you can read the literature and talk about it, the world begins to open up to you.

So I think a solid science base, then genetics. Basic genetics, and then one or more courses in nutrigenomics. You have to be really good at metabolism to get into the nutrition end of genetics. If you want to get into food science, functional food development, or consumer marketing, then you're going to have to take the appropriate courses. There must be a clinical practicum. It can't be "book learning" alone. In addition to the particular skills for your focus area, such as clinical nutrition, you need to learn how to establish a practice, how to run a business, how to talk to the accountant, how to counsel patients concerning genetic information, and how to deal with ethical and legal issues.

So what should we do?

I think we need two tracks. The second one is for retrofitting the practicing dietitian.

EXHIBIT 10–2 *continued*

I'm in favor of Internet-based training components. I've already piloted a course on nutrigenomics for clinical practitioners, and I'm working on developing the practicum training now. You have to have some hands-on experience or this isn't really going to resonate.

I don't have it worked out if it needs to be a Ph.D. or a master's level. I think it's a two-year graduate-level course in nutritional genomics. You cannot stuff all this into the undergraduate program.

We have to get away from training everybody to do everything for everyone. It's too watered down. Our education needs to be hard-core, stand-alone, and respectable or we'll always be in the position of having to prove ourselves. We need to know the transmission of genetics, how a gene goes from generation to generation, plus molecular genetics and molecular nutrition. This then serves as the foundation for developing competency in nutritional genomics, which includes understanding genetic analysis, how to read the results, how to translate them into practical applications, how to provide the needed counseling. Clinical applications will be the first area to hit practice, so the initial focus will be on developing clinically relevant skills— but the other areas of nutritional genomics will be right behind and will need to be addressed as well.

What type of people are needed?

We need people who are really competent. I just can't see the future of dietetics without competency and visibility for that competency. A degree helps, but it's really all about competency and attitude. You have to be able to go toe-to-toe with the physician. It's "You're really good in medicine and I'm really good in nutrition, and if we hook this together, we have a prayer of helping these patients. But neither one of us alone is sufficient." When you get a really good working relationship going, they're thrilled. The synergy is much better than either of you individually and the reward is improved patient care, which they recognize and appreciate once they see it happening.

continues

EXHIBIT 10–2 *continued*

What is the future for genetics in nutrition?

I can't imagine any aspect of dietetics that nutritional genomics isn't going to touch in some way. This includes food science and the development of functional foods. It's the whole food end of things, all the way up to the nutrition intervention. A real plus for us is that we will be able, finally, to intelligently approach health promotion. We're the only healthcare profession that really has the tools for preventing disease. Health care is so complex; it's such a team effort. We need to carve out the nutrition part as something unique. We want to keep our go-getters from going off to some other profession. We have the opportunity to create a whole new sub-discipline for dietetics, or possibly restructure the whole field.

Table 10–1 Example of a Career Ladder Incorporating Advanced Dietetics Practice

	Basic Level of Practice	Specialty Level of Practice	Advanced Level of Practice
Minimum educational level	B.S. plus RD	M.S. in dietetics plus RD	Practice doctorate in dietetics plus RD
Minimum practice experience	1–3 years post-RD experience	More than 3 years post-RD experience	More than 8 years of post-RD experience
Salary increment	Minimum equivalent to median for current ADA salary survey for local area	10% increase over basic level	20% increase over basic level
Clinical expertise	Demonstrates competency in basic practice	Sees a minimum of 100 patients per year to maintain competence in specialty	Sees a minimum of 50 patients per year to maintain competence in specialty
			Attends annual continuing education concerning medications as approved
Clinical privileges	May order supplements and lab tests as specified in approved protocols	May order supplements and lab tests as specified in approved protocols; may reduce texture modifications of diet (e.g., general to soft)	Clinical privileges to adjust nutrients and medications; independently order lab tests; manage fluid and electrolyte status; teach diet,

Table 10–1 Continued

	Basic Level of Practice	Specialty Level of Practice	Advanced Level of Practice
Clinical privileges			insulin, physical activity interaction, and insulin pump use; place feeding tubes; order parenteral and enteral nutrition; conduct genetic testing and related nutrition counseling, as defined within the practice environment
Education	Provides patient education individually and in classes	Provides patient education individually and in classes; serves as a preceptor for dietetics students	Provides patient education individually and in classes; serves as a preceptor for dietetics, nursing, medical, and pharmacy students, residents, and fellows
			Teaches graduate-level classes
Research	Interprets research findings for application to practice; collects data for research protocols	Interprets research findings for application to practice; collects data for research protocol	Interprets research findings for application to practice; collects data for research protocols
		Serves on committees to develop research protocols	Serves as a consultant to committees developing research protocols
		Collaborates on publications in peer-reviewed journals	Serves as the principal investigator for funded studies
			Publishes findings in peer-reviewed journals
Administration	Participates in committees	Participates in multidisciplinary committees	Develops and chairs multidisciplinary committees
	Performs quality management functions	Initiates quality management projects	Develops and implements policies and protocols for patient management implementation
			Develops and implements systems for quality management

(continues)

Table 10-1 Continued

	Basic Level of Practice	Specialty Level of Practice	Advanced Level of Practice
Leadership	Participates in professional organizations	Participates as a leader in professional organizations	Participates as a leader in professional organizations
			Serves as a consultant for standards, guide-lines, and policy de-velopment at the state, national, and international levels

Table 10-2 Example of an Application for Clinical Privileges and Scope of Practice

Application for Scope of Practice and Clinical Privileges for Advanced Practice Registered Dietitians

Name_____

Position _____

Dietetics Degree and School _____

Date of Graduation _____

Dietetics Supervised Practice Program _____

Date of Completion _____

Advanced Degree and School _____

Advanced Degree (Major) _____

Board Certification in Dietetics? Yes_____ No_____

Certificate _____

States Where I Am Currently Licensed _____

****

Table 10-2 Continued

Requested	Verified	List of Clinical Privileges: Dietitian
_____	_____	Performing a nutrition-related physical examination, including measurement of height, weight, length, and body composition for the purpose of identifying nutrition-related deficiencies and monitoring medical nutrition therapy
_____	_____	Taking nutrition/medical/surgical and medication histories
_____	_____	Providing formal, written consultation upon request in the area of medical nutrition therapy
_____	_____	Providing initial and follow-up documentation of services written in the medical record
_____	_____	Taking vital signs and collecting laboratory specimens including phlebotomy
_____	_____	Ordering laboratory tests to include CBC with differential, electrolyte panel, chem 20, vitamin and mineral assays, lipid profiles, serum proteins, and amino acids
_____	_____	Placing, replacing, or manipulating nasogastric or nasointestinal feeding tubes, ordering X rays (abdominal films) to confirm feeding tube placement
_____	_____	Ordering diets, nutritional supplements, and medical foods
_____	_____	Ordering enteral feedings and parenteral nutrition containing insulin and H_2 blockers
_____	_____	Ordering consultations as needed with dentistry, medical specialties, pharmacy, psychiatry, psychology, radiology, and social work
_____	_____	Conducting clinical or outcomes research protocols
_____	_____	Adjusting nutrition-related medications (specify drugs)

I understand that these privileges are extended to me based on a thorough review of my education, training and experience, and demonstrated competence. I understand that if my job duties change, I will need to reapply for clinical privileges. I hereby request the above scope of practice and clinical privileges. I have read and agree to abide by the bylaws of the _____ Medical Center.

Applicant _____ Date _____

The scope of practice and clinical privileges requested above are granted to

Applicant _____
as a member of the staff at _____
_____ located in _____ (city), ____ (state)

Clinical director _____ Date _____
Chief of medical staff _____ Date _____

Table 10–3 Sample of a Policy for Order-Writing Privileges for Advanced Practice Dietitians

Lakeview Medical Center	Date Issued 5/07	Revision Date:	Review Date:
Subject: ORDER WRITING PRIVILEGES FOR MEDICAL NUTRITION THERAPISTS (REGISTERED DIETITIANS)			
Approved		Approved	
Approved		Approved	

Policy

Medical nutrition therapies are ordered by registered dietitians whose credentials have been verified by the medical staff office. Medical nutrition therapy and accompanying monitoring may be ordered by registered dietitians according to clinical privileges on file in the medical staff office. The purposes of this policy are

1. To allow registered dietitians to act in a timely fashion to implement medical nutrition therapy within their approved scope of practice

2. To facilitate patient safety and monitoring of high-risk medical nutrition therapies, especially enteral and parenteral nutrition

3. To improve patient satisfaction

Procedure

1. On receipt of a consult for services, the registered dietitian will obtain a nutrition history, perform a physical examination and write a nutrition assessment in the patient's medical record. The registered dietitian will discuss the plan of care with pertinent staff, including the physician.

2. The registered dietitian will record the orders for nutrition intervention and monitoring in the patient's medical record, verify that the date and time are correct, and record his or her signature, credentials, and pager number at the end of the orders.

3. The nurse, pharmacist, medical technologist, phlebotomist, and other credentialed members of the Lakeview Medical Center (LMS) staff may implement a registered dietitian's order upon receiving it. (See the corresponding policy in the LMS policy and procedure manual, nursing, pharmacy, laboratory, and speech pathology sections.)

4. The registered dietitian is responsible for following the patient for monitoring, tolerance to intervention, and changes in nutrition diagnosis and intervention until the patient is stable and continuity of care is assured, or until discharge from LMS.

5. The registered dietitian is privileged to order nutrition supplements per protocol.

6. The advanced practice registered dietitian may order

   a. Nutrition supplements, including oral supplement beverages and functional and fortified foods

   b. Multiple- or single-dose vitamins and minerals administered orally, via enteral feeding tube, or parenterally

   c. Diets modified in texture, consistency, calorie level, macronutrient composition, and vitamin, mineral, or electrolyte composition

   d. Enteral formulas, including modifying the rate, concentration, or administration schedule, or changing the product

   e. Parenteral formulas, including modified macronutrient, micronutrient, electrolyte, vitamin, and mineral composition

Table 10–3 Continued

f. Medications added to the parenteral nutrients

g. Initiate, change the rate or composition, or discontinue intravenous fluids and electrolytes

h. Enteral and parenteral electrolyte supplementation for patients receiving enteral or parenteral feedings

i. Laboratory data as needed to monitor tolerance and effectiveness of diet, enteral nutrition, and parenteral nutrition

Table 10–4 Sample Collaborative Practice Agreement for an Advanced Practice Dietitian in Diabetes Management

Collaborative Practice Agreement

The intent of this document is to authorize the advanced practice dietitian(s) at the _____ clinic(s) to practice under these protocols without direct supervision. This document sets forth guidelines for collaboration between the supervising physician(s) and the advanced practice dietitian(s).

Development, Revision, and Review

Management protocols are developed collaboratively by the advanced practice dietitian, medical director of the clinic, and supervising physician. These protocols will be reviewed annually and revised as necessary.

The Statement of Approval will be signed by all the above parties initially and annually on the approval date. The Statement of Approval recognizes the collegial relationship between the parties and their intention to follow these protocols. Signature on the Statement of Approval implies approval of all the policies, protocols, and procedures in this document. Advanced practice dietitians and physicians who join the staff mid-year or who cover the practice also signify approval of the protocols. It is the task of the medical director to see that the written approval of all the above parties is obtained.

Setting

The advanced practice dietitian will operate under these protocols at the (Name of Institution)_____ clinics listed below:

Clinic 1: (name and address)

Clinic 2: (name and address)

Supervision

The advanced practice dietitians are authorized to practice under the protocols established in this document without the direct (on-site) supervision or approval of the supervising physicians. Consultation with the supervising physicians or their designated backup is available at all times, either on-site or by telephone when consultation is needed for any reason.

Consultation

The advanced practice dietitians are responsible for providing nutrition services to clients of the (name of clinic or agency). The advanced practice dietitians will provide health promotion, screening, safety instructions, and management of acute episodic illness and stable chronic diseases. Referrals will be made, as needed, to other healthcare providers.

(continues)

Table 10–4 Continued

Physician consultation will be sought for all of the following situations and any others deemed appropriate. Whenever a physician is consulted, a notation to that effect, including the physician's name, must be recorded in the patient's medical record.

Consultation will occur:

· Whenever situations arise that go beyond the intent of the protocols or the competence, scope of practice, or experience of the advanced practice dietitians

· Whenever the patient's condition fails to respond to the management plan within an appropriate time frame, based on the advanced practice dietitian's clinical judgment

· For any uncommon, unfamiliar, or unstable patient condition

· For any patient condition that does not fit the commonly accepted diagnostic pattern for a disease/condition

· For any unexplained physical examination or historical finding or abnormal diagnostic finding

· Whenever a patient requests

· For all emergency situations after initial stabilizing care has been initiated

Medical Records

The advanced practice dietitian is responsible for the complete, **legible** documentation of all patient encounters.

Education and Training

The advanced practice dietitian must possess a valid (State) _____ license, maintain current dietetic registration and be recognized by the American Association of Diabetes Educators as an advanced practitioner in Diabetes Management (BC-ADM).

Evaluation of Clinical Care

Evaluation of the advanced practice dietitian will be provided in the following ways:

· A minimum of a monthly review by the supervising physicians of a minimum of 10% of patient charts. A written record of the review is to be kept.

· Annual evaluation by the supervising physicians based on written criteria.

· Informal evaluation during consultations and case review.

· Periodic chart review as part of chart audits by the Quality Assurance Committee.

Practice Guidelines

The advanced practice dietitians are authorized to diagnose and treat nutrition disorders and related conditions under the following current guidelines (including, but not limited to):

American Diabetes Association. Nutrition recommendations and interventions for diabetes: A position statement of the American Diabetes Association. *Diabetes Care* 2007;30:S48–S65.

Mensing C, Boucher J, Cypress M, Weinger K, Mulcahy K, Barta P, Hosey G, Kopher W, Lasichak A, Lamb B, Mangan M, Norman J, Tanja J, Yauk L, Wisdom K, Adams C. National standards for diabetes self-management education. *Diabetes Care* 2007;30:S96–S103.

American Dietetic Association. Evidence analysis library. Available at www.eatright.org.

International standardized language of nutrition and dietetics. Chicago, IL: American Dietetic Association, 2008.

Other published, accepted sources of medical information, as agreed upon by the collaborating parties and/or identified below:

· OSHA guidelines

· CDC guidelines

Table 10–4 Continued

Collaborating Parties: Statement of Approval

We, the undersigned, agree to the terms of this Collaborative Practice Agreement as set forth in this document.

_____ Medical Director

_____ Supervising Physician

_____ Supervising Physician

_____ Supervising Physician

_____ Advanced Practice Dietitian

_____ Advanced Practice Dietitian

_____ Advanced Practice Dietitian

Approval Date _____

Renewal Date _____

Renewal Date _____

Review with legal counsel prior to signing.

Source: This document was modified extensively from one developed for nurses by Judith C. D. Longworth. Available at http://www.nonpf.com/fpcollabagreesample.htm. Accessed May 27, 2007.

During the interviews we conducted as part of our research, one question asked was "What advice do you have for dietitians who want to develop advanced level practice?" A consensus of answers to this question appears in **Table 10–5.** For many dietitians, implementing an advanced practice role will require breaking new ground. As with any change, some opposition to this expansion of the dietitian's

---

Table 10–5 Overcoming Barriers

Dietitians with expertise in advanced MNT will need skills in overcoming barriers if they are to move forward. The following information provides some thoughts on how to overcome barriers to changes that advance MNT practice.

- It is rare that an idea is accepted the first time it is presented. Be prepared to present the new idea over and over so that people can become comfortable with it.
- Questions and discussion indicate interest in a topic and should not be considered a threat. Anticipate questions and prepare responses to them.
- Anticipate objections from people who have a conservative viewpoint, who act as "gatekeepers," or who have an interest in preserving the status quo. Meet with them in advance to discuss their concerns and acknowledge their objections publicly.
- New initiatives require resources in time and money. Accurately estimate and prepare to state the costs and benefits of new initiatives.
- Prepare to counter "turf" issues with a clear presentation of credentials, including extra training that may be needed. Take the time to read the educational standards, scope of practice, and licensure laws for dietetics and for other professions that may be involved. Be prepared to calmly and unemotionally describe the education and training that dietitians have.
- Prepare to demonstrate how advanced MNT practice does not encroach on practice in other areas. Filling an unfilled niche is easier than filing one that is already occupied by another profession.

responsibilities may be expected. Many advanced practice dietitians are experienced at overcoming barriers, and some of their wisdom appears in **Table 10–6.**

The exercise at the end of the chapter relates to the quote that opened this chapter. It is designed to assist the reader in visioning and developing an advanced practice role.

EXPERIENCES TO TRY

1. Read the interviews with the advanced practice dietitians in Exhibits 10–1 and 10–2. After you have done so, go back and look at the advanced practice model described in Chapter 3. The MNT and nutrition pathophysiology expertise of the interviewees in the exhibits in this chapter is obvious. Can you identify examples of the context and attitude themes? What about scientific inquiry, breadth and balance of perspective, leadership, awareness, and collaboration? What role do you think education played in their career development? What role do you think experience played? How do these roles differ from the role you have now? From the role you envision for yourself in the future?

2. Create an idea for an advanced practice job in your area of practice. Create a page or two of text describing a typical day in this job. Next, think about the knowledge, skills, and experience needed for this job. Write them

---

Table 10–6 Advice from the "Pros" on Becoming an Advanced Practice Dietitian

- Get as much education as possible. Learn all that you can so that when asked, you can perform in a credible fashion. You need experience, but you also need a master's or doctoral degree.
- Create a support system for yourself. It may be composed of colleagues, a mentor or two, family members, or friends. Work with others on the job or through organizations.
- Create a balance between your work and the rest of your life. You can perform at a very high level without sacrificing your family and friends. It's a matter managing your time and priorities.
- Participate in groups rather than working alone. If you are in an isolated situation, access a virtual network of supportive colleagues. Create a "brain trust" of like-minded individuals who are moving forward.
- Stay open to different experiences. It's not a matter of the same one year of experience repeated ten times over; it's a matter of new experiences every year over the course of ten years. Volunteer for projects at work or in organizations that will build your skills in leadership, collaboration, and teamwork, and increase your knowledge.
- Find your passion. This may require more than one try, but we're in a big profession. There are tons of opportunities out there.
- Once you have a vision, set some goals. Create a plan to reach your vision. You'll get there.

down on another page, and organize them according to the themes in the advanced practice model presented in Chapter 3.

3. Identify what else you would need to move into the advanced practice position you described in exercise 2. Do you have an advanced degree in dietetics? Do you have 7 to 10 years of practice experience? Do you have a thorough knowledge in nutrition pharmacology related to your area of practice? Do you read, understand, interpret, explain, and debate MNT research? Can you design an outcomes study that would answer an important question in your area of practice?

4. Once you think about the answers to the questions in exercise 3, think about how you might move toward the goal of an advanced practice position. Can you break it down into one-year increments? Does that seem more manageable? Can you obtain the necessary skills in your current job, or would you need to move into another job or area of practice?

REFERENCE

1. Schlesinger AM Jr. Quoteland. Available at http://www.quoteland.com/search.asp. Accessed May 28, 2007.

Glossary

Accreditation   The voluntary process by which a nongovernmental agency grants a time-limited recognition to an institution, organization, business, or other entity after verifying that it has met predetermined and standardized criteria.

Advanced   Being beyond others in progress or ideas; being beyond the elementary or introductory or greatly developed beyond an initial stage.

Advanced level practitioner   A registered dietitian (RD) who has acquired the expert knowledgebase, complex decision-making skills, and clinical competencies for expanded practice, the characteristics of which are shaped by the context in which the RD practices. Advanced practice is characterized by the integration of a broad range of unique theoretical, research-based, and practical knowledge that occurs as a part of training and experience beyond entry level.

Approach   To make advances, especially in an effort to create a desired result.

Attitude   A mental position or feeling of emotion with regard to a fact or state.

Autonomy   The quality or state of being self-governing.

Awareness   Having or showing realization, perception, or knowledge.

Basic level practice   Synonymous with entry-level practice. Consistent with practice during the first three years following dietetic registration.

Baccalaureate degree   A degree awarded for four years of post-secondary or college-level study.

Balance   The stability produced by even distribution of weight on each of a vertical axis.

Board Certification Board certification in dietetics is granted in recognition of an applicant's documented practice experience and successful completion of an examination in the specialty area. In dietetics, board certification is available in gerontological nutrition, sports dietetics, renal nutrition, pediatric nutrition, and gerontology.

Breadth Something full of width.

Certification A type of credential. Certification is a voluntary process by which nongovernmental entities grant a time-limited recognition to an individual after verifying that the individual has met predetermined standardized criteria.

Certified Diabetes Educator A specialty credential that verifies a certain basic level of knowledge in the field of diabetes.

Certified Nutrition Support Dietitian A specialty credential providing a standard of minimum knowledge deemed appropriate for the practice of the nutrition support dietitian.

Client A person who engages the professional advice or services of another.

Clinical privileges The right of a medical staff member to provide specific patient care services in a manner consistent with his or her licensure, education, and expertise.

Collaboration Working jointly with others or together, especially in an intellectual endeavor.

Commission on Accreditation of Dietetic Education The accrediting agency for education programs that seek to prepare students for careers as registered dietitians or dietetics technicians.

Commission on Dietetic Registration The accrediting agency that protects the public through credentialing processes for dietetics practitioners.

Comprehensive Covering completely or broadly.

Consultation A deliberation among physicians on a case or its treatment.

Creativity The power to create, or having the quality of something created rather than imitated.

Credential An umbrella term for programs including licensure, certification, association, and other forms of recognition.

Dependent practitioners Practitioners who require oversight by another profession; they include registered nurses, dietitians, pharmacists, and physical therapists.

Diagnostic reasoning A formal process consisting of three phases—hypothesis generation, hypothesis testing, and hypothesis closure—that is used to establish a causal relationship.

Dietetics The integration and application of principles derived from the sciences of food, nutrition, management, communication, and biological, physiological, behavioral, and social sciences to achieve and maintain optimal human health.

Discernment   Showing insight and understanding.

Doctor of Philosophy (Ph.D.)   The highest academic degree, which requires mastery of a field of knowledge and demonstrated ability to extend that knowledge by performing scholarly research.

Entry-level practice   Practice during the first three years following dietetic registration.

Environment   The circumstances, objects, or conditions by which one is surrounded.

Evidence-based practice   The conscientious, explicit, and judicious use of the current best evidence in making decisions about the care of individual patients.

Exemplar   A typical or standard specimen.

Experience   Having first-hand knowledge of a particular situation.

Expertise   Having, involving, or displaying special skills or knowledge derived from training or experience.

First professional degree   Completion of the academic requirements for beginning practice in a given profession and demonstration of a level of professional skill beyond that normally required for a bachelor's degree.

Independent practitioners   Practitioners who function without oversight of another profession; they include physicians, dentists, veterinarians, and podiatrists.

Initiative   At one's own discretion; independently of outside influence or control.

Integrated   To unite with something else or to incorporate into a larger unit.

Leadership   The capacity to lead.

Licensure   Statutes that include an explicitly defined scope of practice and make performance of the profession illegal without first obtaining a license from the state.

Master's degree   A degree awarded for successful completion of one or two years of full-time, college-level study beyond the baccalaureate degree; it denotes mastery of a particular subject area.

Medical nutrition therapy (MNT)   Nutrition diagnostic, therapeutic, and counseling services for the purpose of disease management that are furnished by a registered dietitian or nutrition professional; a specific application of the nutrition care process in clinical settings that is focused on the management of disease.

Mid-level practitioner   An individual practitioner, other than a physician, dentist, veterinarian, or podiatrist, who is licensed, registered, or otherwise permitted by the United States or the jurisdiction in which he or she practices to dispense a controlled substance in the course of professional practice. Examples of mid-level practitioners include, but are not limited to, healthcare providers such as nurse practitioners, nurse midwives, nurse anesthetists, clinical nurse specialists, and physician assistants who are authorized to dispense controlled substances by the state in which they practice.

Networking A means of exchanging information or services among individuals, groups, or institutions.

Nutrition assessment The systematic process of obtaining, verifying, and interpreting data so as to make decisions about the nature and cause of nutrition-related problems.

Nutrition Care Process A four step problem solving method used by dietitians to identify a diagnosis which drives nutrition intervention, nutrition monitoring, and nutrition evaluation.

Nutrition counseling A supportive process, characterized by a collaborative counselor–patient/client relationship, to set priorities, establish goals, and create individualized action plans that acknowledge and foster responsibility for self-care to treat an existing condition and promote health.

Nutrition diagnosis The process of identifying and labeling an actual occurrence, risk of, or potential for developing a nutritional problem that a dietetics professional is responsible for treating independently.

Nutrition evaluation The systematic comparison of current findings with previous status, intervention goals, or a reference standard.

Nutrition intervention A purposefully planned action designed with the intent of changing a nutrition-related behavior, risk factor, environmental condition, or other aspect of health status for an individual (and his or her family or caregivers), a target group, or the community at large.

Nutrition monitoring The review and measurement of the patient/client/group's status at a scheduled (preplanned) follow-up point with regard to the nutrition diagnosis, intervention, plans/goals, and outcomes.

Nutrition outcomes research The rigorous determination of what works in nutrition care and what does not.

Nutrition pathophysiology The study of suffering related to nutrition.

Nutrition pharmacology The process of balancing nutrient intake and drug doses so as to optimize the therapeutic effect of both nutrients and drugs and thereby improve the health of the patient.

Nutrition prescription The patient/client's individualized recommended dietary intake of energy and/or selected foods or nutrients based on current reference standards and dietary guidelines and the patient/client's health condition and nutrition diagnosis.

Patient An individual under medical care and treatment.

Pattern recognition A complex mental process requiring rapid retrieval of an appropriate match for the diagnosis based on salient clues.

Practice The continuous exercise of a profession.

Practitioner   One who practices a profession.

Prescription   An order for medication that is dispensed to or for an ultimate user. A prescription is *not* an order for medication that is dispensed for immediate administration to the ultimate user (e.g., an order to dispense a drug to an inpatient for immediate administration in a hospital is not a prescription). To be valid, a prescription for a controlled substance must be issued for a legitimate medical purpose by a practitioner acting in the usual course of sound professional practice. A medical prescription is an order (often in written form) from a qualified healthcare professional to a pharmacist or other therapist for a treatment to be provided to the patient. A prescription is a legal document that not only instructs the dispenser in the preparation and provision of the medicine or device, but also indicates that the prescriber takes responsibility for the clinical care of the patient and the outcomes that may or may not be achieved.

Profession   An occupation that requires extensive training and the study and mastery of specialized knowledge, and usually has a professional association, ethical code, and process of certification or licensing.

Referral   The act of sending a patient to another health professional. It may also refer to the document authorizing a visit with a health professional.

Registration   The least restrictive form of state regulation. As with certification, unregistered persons may be permitted to practice the profession if they do not use the state-recognized title. Typically, exams are not given and enforcement of the registration requirement is minimal.

Regulation   A legal restriction promulgated by government administrative agencies through rule making supported by a threat of sanction or a fine.

Risk   A factor likely to result in adverse consequences.

Scientific inquiry   An examination into facts or principles.

Scope of practice   A description of the range of services that a professional is authorized to provide.

Sign   Objective evidence of disease, especially as observed and interpreted by the physician rather than by the patient or lay observer.

Simplified   Reduced to basic essentials.

Socratic method   A vehicle used to analyze a given situation, consider the possibilities, and derive a clear argument supporting the desired outcome.

Specialization   Concentrating or delimiting one's focus to part of the whole field of dietetics (such as ambulatory care, long-term care, diabetes, renal, pediatric, private practice, community, nutrition support, research, or sports nutrition).

Specialty practice   Concentrating or delimiting one's focus to part of the whole field of dietetics.

Statutory certification   A type of certification that limits the use of particular titles to persons meeting predetermined requirements; persons who are not certified could still practice the occupation or profession, however.

Symptom   Subjective evidence of disease or physical disturbance observed by the patient.

Index